Acid
and
Alkaline

by Herman Aihara

George Ohsawa Macrobiotic Foundation
Oroville, California

By Herman Aihara

Acid and Alkaline
Basic Macrobiotics
Kaleidoscope
Learning From Salmon
Macrobiotics: An Invitation to
  Health and Happiness
Milk – A Myth of Civilization
Seven Macrobiotic Principles

First Edition	1971
Revised Edition	1977
Third Edition	1980
Fourth Edition	1982
Fifth Edition	1986

George Ohsawa Macrobiotic Foundation
1511 Robinson Street, Oroville, California 95965

ISBN 0-918860-44-x

Preface

"East is East and West is West and never the twain shall meet," said Rudyard Kipling. He lived in the Orient too soon. If he lived there now his opinion would be much different.

Judo, karate and other martial arts have thousands of students and are important sports in the Western world: they will be practiced even at the elementary level in the near future. They have a different spirit than football or baseball. They are aiming more at spiritual than physical development. The West is learning something from the East.

Japan learned how to make the automobile, camera, transistor, etc., from the West. Its industry was built with Eastern spirit, adding Western technology. Japan's products are now so superb that one of the largest auto makers in the West is dying.

East and West have met and are creating a tremendous civilization. This will be realized in the 21st century. It is starting already. Judo, Aiki, Zen, Yoga, television, and transistors are the first stage of such a civilization. At the fifth and sixth stages of judgment, East and West will meet at the religious and conceptual levels. This will be very difficult. When they merge, one world will be established.

My purpose in writing this book is to guide the general public of the West to accept the Eastern concept of science and apply it to Western thought in medicine. This will be a great benefit for our health.

Herman Aihara
November, 1979

iii

This book is dedicated to my teachers at elementary school, high school, and the University; to George Ohsawa and Lima-san; to my father and mother and my adoptive parents; to my brother-in-law; and to the many authors whose works inspired me to write this book.

Herman Aihara
February 20, 1980

Contents

CHAPTER I

The Importance of Acid and Alkaline Balance

1. Why this Book was Written

From the end of the last century to this century, important concepts of life were brought to the field of physiology. One of them is *milieu interne*, brought forward by Claude Bernard. Another is *homeostasis*, by Walter Cannon. "Claude Bernard, the great nineteenth century physiologist who originated much of our modern physiological thought, called the extracellular fluids that surround the cells the *milieu interne*, 'the internal environment,' and Walter Cannon, another great physiologist of the first half of this century, referred to the maintenance of constant conditions in these fluids as *homeostasis*." (Guyton, *Function of the Human Body*.) In this homeostasis, our body has to maintain many constant conditions. That is to say:

1. The body temperature (98.6° F.)
2. Acidity and alkalinity of the body fluids (pH 7.4)
3. The concentration of certain chemicals dissolved in the body fluids
4. The glucose level in the blood
5. The amount of body fluids
6. The levels of O_2 and CO_2 in the blood
7. The amount of blood. . . etc.

Dr. Cannon realized the importance of balance between acid and alkaline in the body fluids, especially in the blood. Although Western medicine or physiology developed the theory of how our body maintains the balance of acid and alkaline in our blood, which should be maintained slightly on the alkaline side, it didn't develop this concept further into the nutritional field.

Around the same time of Dr. Cannon, a distinguished medical doctor lived in Japan. Dr. Tan Katase, who was a professor at Osaka University, devoted his whole life to the study of calcium, its physiological dietary function and importance in human health. He studied physiology with an eye to human health. One of his conclusions was the same as that of Dr. Cannon's, but since Dr. Katase was interested more in health than in mere physiology, he related the acid and alkaline balance to foods. He recommended highly alkaline foods containing calcium.

A little before Dr. Katase, there lived in Japan an army doctor by the name of Sagen Ishizuka, who concluded after twenty-eight years of experience and study as an army doctor that two alkaline elements in our body fluid serve important functions for health. According to him, the two alkaline elements determine the character of foods, and likewise determine the character in men who eat such foods. Those two elements are potassium and sodium.

His disciple, George Ohsawa, cured his own 'incurable' sickness by Ishizuka's diet. He then developed Ishizuka's theory further and called it the macrobiotic diet. (In Greek, *macro* means great or long, and *bio* means life.) Ohsawa applied Oriental philosophy to the acid and alkaline concept, and called them yin and yang, which are the basic and most popular concepts in Oriental thought.

In my studies, I have found that *foods* can be very well

organized if they are classified by the two pairs of balancing concepts, acid/alkaline and yin/yang. In this book I am trying to unite the Western concept of acid and alkaline and the Eastern concept of yin and yang, because when these concepts are combined our health will be benefitted very much. For example, cancer will be better understood using these concepts of acid and alkaline and yin and yang. And these concepts can give a better approach to the cancer-curing diet. The concepts of yin and yang benefit not only our health; they also open vast fields of Oriental thought which will add a deeper psychological and spiritual understanding of life to the Westerner. By the same token, the concepts of acid and alkaline will give the Easterner a better understanding of life and better guide toward health. This book was written with these benefits in mind.

2. Immortality

Since ancient times people have searched for immortality; in Europe, chemistry was developed as the result. In China, medicine was developed.

Theoretically, we are immortal. Egg and sperm combine and create new cells. From these new cells, new life develops. This new life makes egg and sperm, again forming new life. In other words, germ cells never die. Parents live on and on in new life.

Eggs and sperm are germ cells. According to modern physiology (*Man and the Living World*), germ cells do not show signs of age, and carry the potential of life from generation to generation. However, we have other kinds of cells which are body cells or somatic cells. As they grow, these cells turn into specialized tissue such as nerve, muscle, connective tissue, tendon, cartilage, skin, bone, fatty tissue, etc. These tissues grow further to become specialized organs. These specialized cells of tissues and organs unfortunately reach old age and die. What makes these cells die?

A famous French physiologist, Alexis Carrel, found the cause. He kept a chicken heart alive for about twenty-eight years. He incubated a chicken egg. The heart of the developing young chick was taken out and cut in pieces. These, consisting of many cells, were transferred into a saline solution which contained minerals in the same proportion as chicken blood. He changed this solution every day, and kept the chick's heart alive about twenty-eight years. When he stopped changing this solution, the heart died. What made the chick's heart stay alive?

The secret of why Carrel's chick heart survived twenty-eight years lies in the fact that he changed the fluid in which the chick's heart was kept, every day. Carrel's experiment brought us to modern physiology, which says:

> For the cells of the body to continue living, there is one major requirement: the composition of the body fluids that bathe the outside of the cells must be controlled very exactly from moment to moment and day to day, with no single important constituent ever varying more than a few percent. Indeed, cells can live even after being removed from the body if they are placed in a fluid bath that contains the same constituents and has the same physical conditions as those of the body fluids. Claude Bernard . . . called the extracellular fluids that surround the cells the *milieu interne,* 'the internal environment,' and Walter Cannon . . . referred to the maintenance of constant conditions in these fluids as *homeostasis.*
>
> (Guyton, *Function of the Human Body.*)

Then why does the environmental fluid have to be kept in a constant condition? What kind of relation is there between cells, organs, and body fluids? In order to answer these questions we have to go back billions of years to the origin of life.

3. Origin of Life – Water

No living thing, whether living in water or on land, can live without water. No single body cell can sustain life without water. Therefore, the most accepted biological theory of creation is that life started in the ocean. It is interesting to note that the Chinese ideogram for the sea (海) is made up of three parts:

Water (氵)   Man (人)   and Mother (母).

This ideogram means that the sea is the mother of man. In the beginning, unicellular structures emerged from an ocean which nourished them – probably about three billion years ago.

This ocean was a perfect environment for the primitive unicellular organisms because the specific heat of water is very great. This means that the ocean temperature is only minutely affected by weather, climate, and location. Furthermore, water is a strong solvent. Therefore, it can contain almost all the nutrients that living creatures require.

Then, due to the change of weather and foods eaten, some single-celled creatures transformed into more complicated multicellular organisms. When this happened, the organisms had to carry the ocean between the cells and inside the cells, because some of the cells were not in contact with the outside ocean; that means they had no foods to get, and no waste to throw out. By bringing the ocean inside, the multicellular organisms could live in the ocean in the same way the unicellular organism lived, because the 'internal ocean' was the same composition as the outside ocean. Today, however, the ocean is much saltier than our extracellular fluid because ocean water became saltier during billions of years of evaporation. The present ocean is so salty that we cannot even use it for drinking water. If we drink this ocean water, it will increase the osmotic pressure until we lose our inside liquid, dehydrate, and die. Osmotic pressure is very important for keeping the amount of water constant in our body. This osmotic pressure is due to the fact that water has a strong soluble power.

The next important chemical characteristic of water is ionization. Ionization happens when an atom loses its electrons or gains electrons from another atom. This happens in a water solution. For example, when salt (sodium chloride, NaCl) dissolves in water, chlorine (Cl) acquires electrons from the sodium (Na) atom and becomes a negatively charged atom. [This is called minus (–) or negative ionization.] On the other hand, when Na loses its electron it becomes a positively charged atom. This is called positive ionization.

Since ionized elements activate reactions, elements which cause chemical reactions are generally considered ionized. Since water causes ionization, without water our body ceases its chemical reactions. This means death.

The transformation to multicellular organisms was a big change in life, because in multicellular organisms individual cells began to specialize. Some became sterile and functioned only through locomotion and food acquisition, while others retained the primitive condition of the reproductive cell. Some of the reproductive cells became highly specialized (egg and sperm) while others merely retained their initial capacity to reproduce by simple fission. In other words, a differentiation of function took place among the cells of the aggregate, definitely distinguishing it from the isolated single cells, and at the same time creating the first step in the organization of a complex animal through the loss of reproductive power. Once this step was taken, differentiation of the soma cells continued in various directions toward greater and greater complexity, and then up the long trail to a highly intricate form such as man.

Another important change that resulted in multicellular organisms was that they began to carry the outside environment (the ocean) inside of their bodies, as I said in a previous paragraph. These multicellular cells were shut off from any chance of directly obtaining food, water, and oxygen from the distant larger environment or from discharging into it the waste materials which result from activity. The conveniences for getting supplies and eliminating debris were provided by the development of moving streams within the body itself: the blood and tissue fluids. By building circulatory systems, living creatures acquired much more freedom than single-celled organisms and developed into the more complicated creatures known as fish.

Some of the more yang (I will explain this word later) fish developed the ability to utilize oxygen from the air and not from the water. They became amphibians. Emerging from water to land was the second biggest change in animal life. As the new environment changed its temperature, moisture, and oxygen contents, food conditions changed qualitatively and quantitatively. The variation of environmental conditions and foods developed the complexity of the body structure and function of specialized animal cells, resulting in highly developed muscles, organs, coordinating nervous and glandular systems including digestive organs, circulatory organs, respiratory organs, and poison eliminating and waste control organs. As a result, animals could maintain steadier inner conditions than before; they were provided with coordinated nervous and glandular systems.

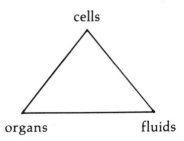

Organs, the fluid inner environment, and cells were dependent on each other. For the multicellular organisms and higher living creatures, it seems to me these three are dependent on each other. If one of them malfunctions or becomes rotten, the others will die. However, for the simplest creatures, unicellular organisms, fluids were originally outside, and that was the origin of cells. The condition and constitution of fluid produced the first cell. (This is not an orthodox biological theory today; only a few biologists believe this, including Dr. K. Chishima.)

Therefore, in my opinion, the condition and constitution of body fluid, especially blood, is the most important factor in our life: that is to say, for our health. In man, organs such as the kidneys, liver, and especially the large intestine eliminate waste and toxins and maintain our internal environment in as ideal a condition as possible. However, there is limitation for this. If we eat too many poison-producing foods, or not enough materials which are needed to clear out poisons, then our internal environment becomes beyond control, and away from the correct condition in which our cells can live. The cells become sick and die. Many sicknesses are a function of the body's attempt to clean up this internal environment. Cancer is a condition in which body cells become abnormal due to the abnormal condition of body fluids.

Then what should be the condition of body fluids, including the blood? That is to say, what should be the balance of acidity and alkalinity? The body fluid should be slightly alkaline, as Dr. Walter Cannon pointed out: "It is of the greatest importance to the existence and proper action of the cells that the blood shall not vary to a noteworthy degree either in the acid or the alkaline direction." This applies also to the extracellular fluids.

Now I will discuss acid and alkaline.

4. What the Study of Acid and Alkaline Will Do for You

When they are metabolized, carbohydrates, proteins, and fats produce inorganic and organic acids. Protein produces sulfuric acid and phosphoric acid. Carbohydrates and fats produce acetic acid and lactic acid. These acids are all poisonous. We have to eliminate them from our bodies as quickly as possible. However, if these acidic substances were eliminated through the kidneys and large intestine, those organs would suffer damage from the acid. Luckily, however, in our body those acids are neutralized by mineral compounds. Together, the mineral compounds and acids produce substances which are no longer poisonous to us and which can be safely eliminated.

The family of mineral compounds which neutralize acids are the carbonic salts, symbolized as $BaCO_3$ where the Ba stands for any one of the four basic or alkaline elements: Na, Ca, K, and Mg. When carbonic salts meet with strong acids such as sulfuric acid, phosphoric acid, acetic acid, and lactic acid, the alkaline minerals making up the carbonic salt leave the salt and combine with the acids to make new salts. For example:

$$BaCO_3 + H_2SO_4 = BaSO_4 + H_2O + CO_2$$

carbonic salt + sulfuric acid = sulfuric salt + water + carbon dioxide.

In the result, carbonic salt changes sulfuric acid, which is a strong acid, to sulfuric salt, which can be eliminated through the kidneys without any harm. In the same way, some other acid may be changed to another salt and be eliminated through the wall of the large intestine. In short, the acids which are the end product of metabolism can be eliminated *only* after they are changed to neutral salts. Then they are no longer harmful to the kidneys and to the wall of the intestine.

The result of this change, that is to say, from acid to neutral salt is to reduce the concentration of alkaline elements such as Na, Ca, Mg, and K in the blood and then in the extracellular fluid. It is this lowered concentration of alkaline elements which is referred to as the acidic condition of the body fluid. Since in order for us to be healthy our body fluid must be kept at an alkaline level (pH 7.4), we must re-supply the lost alkaline elements through the foods we eat.

This is one of the reasons that we have to eat enough alkaline forming foods to make body fluids alkaline all the time. Another reason that we have to eat alkaline forming foods is that a shortage of the alkaline forming elements Na and Ca in the extracellular fluids causes a lowering of the other alkaline forming elements, K and Mg, in the intracellular fluids of the body. If the intracellular fluids in question are in nerve cells, then the nerves will not function; that is to say, the nerves will not transmit messages. The result is that we go into a coma. Therefore, it is imperative to keep enough alkaline forming elements in our body fluids to maintain an alkalinity level of pH 7.4.

Furthermore, one of the important causes of cancer – and other degenerative diseases – is the cumulative effect of the acidic condition of body fluid. Therefore if you study acid and alkaline balance as taught in this book, you can prevent almost all sicknesses, including cancer, heart disease, heart attack, and AIDS.

CHAPTER II

Acid and Alkaline – The Western Approach

1. Acid and Alkaline in the Household

You find acid in your car. The liquid contained in the battery is acid. Actually, this is strong acid – sulfuric acid. If the liquid drops on your clothes, it will burn. This liquid tastes sour.

A meaning of the word *acid* is sour, sharp, or biting to the taste. The sour taste of oranges, grapefruit, grapes, or sour milk is due to acids which they contain. We cannot distinguish an acid by its appearance. There is a convenient and simple means of detecting acidity. This is done with litmus paper. Litmus is a blue vegetable compound extracted from lichens, and its color changes to red when it comes in contact with an acid. You can buy litmus paper at most drug stores. It is an absorbent paper which has been dipped in a litmus solution and dried. It comes in strips and there are two kinds: blue and red. The blue type is for detecting acids and the red is for alkaline detection.

Pour a small amount of vinegar into a tumbler and dip a strip of blue litmus paper in it. The blue color will change to red. Acid in the vinegar has caused the change in color. Vinegar is principally a weak solution of acetic acid. Acetic acid is used commercially for making the compounds called acetates. Photographic film, some artificial silks, some plastics and enamels are acetates. Wash the tumbler which contained the vinegar and squeeze some lemon juice into it. Blue litmus paper will turn red because lemon juice contains citric acid.

Many food substances other than lemon juice and vinegar contain acids which can be detected with blue litmus paper. Dip pieces of blue litmus paper into a number of wet foods such as grapefruit juice, tomato juice, sour milk, etc., and see the reaction of the litmus paper.

There is considerable tannic acid in tea and coffee. Tannic acid is also called tannin. You can detect its presence in these beverages with blue litmus paper.

Lye, baking soda, and soap, when dissolved in water, produce compounds which are alkaline. The alkalines, like the acids, show their characteristics only when in a water solution. A dry alkaline or a dry acid is inactive. Generally, an alkaline turns red litmus paper to blue. Why does alkaline turn red litmus paper blue? Pour a small amount of household ammonia into a tumbler and dip a strip of red litmus paper in it. The red litmus will turn blue. Lime, water, or milk of magnesia turn red litmus paper blue.

When an acid and an alkaline are mixed together there is an immediate reaction. They neutralize each other and when this happens the alkaline and the acid both disappear. In their place appears water and a compound called a salt. The word 'salt' as commonly used refers to the sodium chloride used in cooking. But in chemistry, salt is the general name of a large group of useful compounds. The following are salts found in the household:

Common Name	Chemical Name
salt	sodium chloride
baking soda	sodium bicarbonate
borax	sodium tetraborate
soap	sodium stearate
plaster of Paris	calcium sulfate
chalk	calcium carbonate

The soil, especially in dark, shady places where moss is growing, often contains enough acid to turn blue litmus paper red. To check the acidity or alkalinity of soil, mix it with water and dip a strip of litmus paper into it. If it turns red litmus to blue, the soil is alkaline. If blue litmus turns red in the solution, the soil is acid.

Generally speaking, the metabolic process of the plant world is from acid to alkaline, while the metabolic process of the animal world is from alkaline to acid.

2. What Are Acids and Alkalies?

According to Funk and Wagnall's Encyclopedia:

> Acids are chemical compounds containing the element hydrogen, and having the ability to supply positively charged hydrogen ions to a chemical reaction. Acidity is a relative term, depending upon the comparative ability to donate or accept hydrogen ions. Thus water, which is ordinarily considered neutral, acts as an alkaline substance when dissolved in pure acetic acid, and as an acid when dissolved in liquid ammonia. . . .
>
> Most acids are characterized by sour taste, specific action on certain organic dyes (notably the reddening of blue litmus), the ability to dissolve certain metals (such as zinc) with the liberation of hydrogen, and the ability to neutralize alkaline substances.
>
> Alkalies are a class of chemical compounds, also called bases, which have the property of forming the ion OH⁻ in solution. Their properties are generally opposite to those of acids, and they neutralize acids, reacting with them to form salts. The term was originally applied to the salts obtained by leaching the ashes of plants, consisting chiefly of the carbonates of sodium and potassium, but it is now usually restricted to the hydroxides of *alkali*

metals, lithium, sodium, potassium, rubidium, cesium, francium, and of the radical ammonium, NH_4. . . . The alkalies are all soluble in water, as also are most of the compounds of the alkali metals. The alkali metals are all monovalent, and are strongly electropositive.

Atoms have protons in their centers (nuclei) and electrons in their orbits, as illustrated.

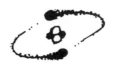

In 1913, Neils Bohr, a Danish scientist, suggested an atomic model which serves chemists well to the present day. E. L. Rutherford established that the atom's mass is concentrated in the infinitesimally small nucleus, which carries a positive electrical charge. Circling around the nucleus in never-ending orbits are clusters of negatively charged satellites called electrons. The negative charge of the orbital electrons is offset by the positive charge of the nucleus, so that the atom, in its normal state, is electrically neutral.

In the case of normal hydrogen (H), the atom is a proton circled by an electron, as shown in the illustration above. If the hydrogen atom loses this electron, then only the proton remains; this is called a hydrogen ion (H^+). Since this is not a normal state for the hydrogen atom, it is chemically unstable, or active. This proton (H^+) stimulates our tongue and causes the sour taste. The chemical solution causing this sour taste is called acid. Compounds which combine with protons are called alkaline; they have an extra electron such as OH⁻.

In our body fluids – blood and cell fluid – acid and alkaline change from one to the other and always maintain a constant condition of alkalinity or acidity. Acid and alkaline are the front and back of one coin, a chemical property of any solution.

3. Acid and Alkaline in the Human Body

Our body secretes or maintains many different kinds of fluids. Their pH factors are different. The most important of these fluids is blood, which has to be slightly alkaline all the time.

Table 1. Sample pH Values

Acid	pH	Alkaline	pH
stomach juice	1.5	saliva	7.1
wine	3.5	blood	7.4
beer	4.4	sea water	8.1
cow's milk	6.5	pancreatic juice	8.8
		soap	9.1
		baking soda	12.0

Our body's exercises or movements produce lactic acid and carbon dioxide. In water, carbon dioxide becomes carbonic acid. Phosphoric acid and sulfuric acid are likewise produced in the body from the oxidation of the phosphorus and sulfur contained in food. This makes the blood acid. On the other hand, alkaline elements such as sodium, potassium, magnesium, and calcium are ingested in large amounts, especially in vegetable food. The gastric juices secreted to digest the alkaline foods are acid. The blood acidity is reduced with the secretion of bile which is alkaline and with the high intake of alkaline forming vegetable food, making the blood alkaline.

The degree of acidity in a solution depends on the number of hydrogen ions (H^+) present. Similarly, the degree of alkalinity in a solution depends on the concentration of the combined elements hydrogen (H) and oxygen (O), to which has been added a free electron causing a negative charge; this is called a hydroxyl ion (OH^-).

In pure water at 22°C. there is one gram of ionic hydrogen in ten thousand liters of water, or the hydrogen concentration is one ten-millionth or $1/10^7$ or 10^{-7}. In pure water, the hydroxyl ion concentration is also 10^{-7}. It is customary to use pH=7 to denote this concentration of hydrogen ions. If the hydrogen ion concentration of a solution is 10^{-6}, then the pH is 6. This shows the acid concentration of the solution. If the hydrogen ion concentration is 10^{-8}, then the pH is 8. Thus if the pH is larger than 7, the solution is alkaline. If it is smaller than 7, the solution is acid.

The pH of blood is 7.4. This means that it is slightly alkaline. This alkalinity has to be kept almost constant; even minor variations are dangerous. If the hydrogen ion concentration in the blood rises to pH 6.95 (barely over the line on the acid side), coma and death result. And, if the hydrogen ion concentration in the blood falls from pH 7.4 to pH 7.7, tetanic convulsions occur. With acid blood, the heart relaxes and ceases to beat, and with too alkaline blood it contracts and ceases to beat.

Two compounds are dissolved in our blood plasma. One is sodium bicarbonate ($NaHCO_3$) (alkaline) and the other is carbonic acid (H_2CO_3) (volatile acid). If we increase the amount of carbonic acid, as in exercise, the blood becomes more acid. But if we breathe deeply and rapidly for a minute or two, the concentration of CO_2 in the alveoli of the lungs is lowered, causing the lungs to remove CO_2 from the blood. That means the H_2CO_3 in the blood loses CO_2 and becomes H_2O. Thus the blood becomes less acid and more alkaline.

Another way the body prevents increased acidity is through blood buffers. Blood buffers are mixtures of weak acids and salts of strong bases. Blood buffers work to keep the pH from fluctuating in extreme, and resist changes in hydrogen ion concentration. More about blood buffers (from Cannon, *The Wisdom of the Body*):

> If a non-volatile acid, such as hydrochloric acid (HCl) or lactic acid, which we may symbolize as HL, is added to the blood, it unites with some of the sodium of the sodium bicarbonate and drives off carbon dioxide, according to the following equations:
>
> $$HCl + NaHCO_3 = NaCl + H_2O + CO_2 \text{ or}$$
> $$HL + NaHCO_3 = NaL + H_2O + CO_2$$
>
> [*Note: NaL, which is alkaline, is the transformation of HL, acid.*]
>
> The NaCl is common table salt, a neutral, harmless substance. The H_2O and CO_2 form the familiar carbonic acid (H_2CO_3), which is volatile. The addition of the strong acid, HCl or HL, has, to be sure, made the blood temporarily more acid by increasing the carbonic acid. As we have already learned, however, the increase of CO_2 stimulates the respiratory center, and the consequent increased ventilation of the lungs quickly and readily gets rid of the extra acid - both that produced by displacement from $NaHCO_3$ as in the equations above and that which is now in excess because the $NaHCO_3$ has been reduced. As soon as the extra carbon dioxide

is pumped out, and the usual ratio H_2CO_3 to $NaHCO_3$ gradually returns, the normal reaction of the blood is restored and the deeper breathing stops.

In the circumstances described in the foregoing paragraphs, the sodium bicarbonate of the plasma served to protect the blood from any considerable change in the acid direction. Because of its capacity to perform that function, it is called a 'buffer' salt. Another buffer salt present in the blood, especially in the red blood corpuscles, is alkaline sodium phosphate (Na_2HPO_4). When acid is added to blood, not only is it 'buffered' by sodium bicarbonate, but also by the alkaline sodium phosphate, as shown in the following equation:

$$Na_2HPO_4 + HCl = NaH_2PO_4 + NaCl$$

Again note that common salt (NaCl) is formed, and also acid (dihydrogen) sodium phosphate. It happens that both the 'alkaline' and the 'acid' sodium phosphate are almost neutral substances. The strong hydrochloric acid, in the change symbolized in the equation, has, therefore, not altered the reaction of the blood to an important degree by transforming the alkaline into the acid form of the phosphate. The acid phosphate has, however, a slightly acid reaction and it must not be permitted to accumulate in the fluid matrix. Unlike carbonic acid, it is non-volatile and therefore cannot be breathed away. Here the kidney plays its part in restricting the oscillations of the acid and the alkali of the blood.

If large amounts of non-volatile – and consequently non-respirable – acid appear in the blood, there is danger that the fixed bases of the blood salts, especially sodium, may be carried away through the kidneys and thus lost from the body. In this condition, it is interesting to note that ammonia (NH_3), which is alkaline, can be used to neutralize the acid in place of sodium. Ammonia is a waste product of organic processes, which is ordinarily transformed into the neutral substance, urea, and eliminated. Whenever loss of the fixed bases, e.g., sodium, calcium and potassium, is threatened, ammonium salts are formed and discharged into the blood, then filtered out through the glomeruli and the kidney tubules.

4. The Newer Theory of Acid and Alkaline

The newer theory of acid and alkaline defines acid as any substance that gives protons (H^+ ions), and an alkali as any substance that combines with protons. Acids are proton donors, and alkalies are proton receptors.

This definition of an acid is equivalent to the older view, but the definition of an alkali is much broader in its implications. The following equations will clarify the point:

	Acid		Alkaline
1)	HCl	$\leftrightarrow$	$H^+ + Cl^-$
2)	HCN	$\leftrightarrow$	$H^+ + CN^-$
3)	CH_3COOH	$\leftrightarrow$	$H^+ + CH_3COO^-$
4)	H_2CO_3	$\leftrightarrow$	$H^+ + HCO_3^-$
5)	HCO_3	$\leftrightarrow$	$H^+ + CO_3^-$
6)	H_2SO_4	$\leftrightarrow$	$H^+ + HSO_4^-$
7)	HSO_4	$\leftrightarrow$	$H^+ + SO_4^-$
8)	NH_4	$\leftrightarrow$	$H^+ + NH_3^-$
9)	NH_3	$\leftrightarrow$	$H^+ + NH_2^-$
10)	H_2O	$\leftrightarrow$	$H^+ + OH^-$
11)	H_3O	$\leftrightarrow$	$H^+ + H_2O^-$

According to the new concept of acid and alkaline, water and ammonia can be either acid or alkaline. This is shown in the following examples:

1) In equation 10, water gives H^+, so it is acid.
2) In equation 11, water accepts H^+, so it is alkaline.
3) In equation 9, ammonia gives H^+, so it is acid.
4) In equation 8, ammonia accepts H^+, so it is alkaline.

In conclusion, acid and alkaline are the two characteristic conditions of a solution. Any solution is either more acid or more alkaline. If acidic characteristics dominate, the solution is acid. However, there is no absolute acid or alkaline. An acid solution always contains some alkaline factors, and an alkaline solution always contains some acid factors. Neutrality is an ideal condition in which the amount of acid (H^+) and alkalinity (OH^-) is equal. It is an ideal state, and not realistic. In reality, what we eat or drink is always more acid or alkaline.

The characteristics of acid and alkaline are very similar to the Oriental concept of yin and yang. This appears in ancient great Chinese books such as the *Tao Te Ching* and the *Nei Ching*. The concept of yin and yang is the concept of life. They are not static: yin and yang conditions are always changing in our life, exactly as acid and alkaline works in us. I see here the similarity between the Western concept of chemistry or life – acid and alkaline – and the Eastern concept of life – yin and yang. Acid and alkaline can be defined quantitatively, whereas yin and yang is difficult to express quantitatively; rather it is philosophical. Therefore, it is understandable that Westerners who are more materialistic thinkers developed the acid and alkaline concept and Easterners who are more spiritual thinkers developed the yin yang concept. It is important for us, however, to understand both concepts with equal weight in order to be healthy. In this book I have tried to combine both concepts.

Table 2. pH Values of Various Foods

Food	pH	Food	pH	Food	pH
limes	1.9	sauerkraut	3.5	asparagus	5.6
lemons	2.3	cherries	3.6	cheese	5.6
cranberries	2.5	olives	3.7	potatoes	5.8
gooseberries	2.9	apricots	3.8	wheat flour	6.0
plums	2.9	fruit jam	3.8	tuna	6.0
vinegar	2.9	pears	3.8	peas	6.1
soft drinks	3.0	grapes	4.0	salmon	6.2
apples	3.1	tomatoes	4.2	butter	6.3
cider	3.1	beer	4.5	corn	6.3
fruit jellies	3.1	bananas	4.6	dates	6.3
grapefruit	3.2	pumpkin	5.0	oysters	6.4
sour pickles	3.2	carrots	5.1	cow's milk	6.5
rhubarb	3.2	beets	5.2	maple syrup	6.8
strawberries	3.3	squash	5.2	shrimp	6.9
wine	3.3	cabbage	5.3	pure water	7.0
blackberries	3.4	turnips	5.4	hominy	7.4
dill pickles	3.4	spinach	5.4	salt	7.5
raspberries	3.4	beans	5.5	sodium	7.5
oranges	3.5	white bread	5.5		
peaches	3.5	sweet potatoes	5.5		

5. Acid and Alkaline Forming Elements

There are two types of acid and alkaline foods. One is acid or alkaline foods; the other is acid or alkaline *forming* foods.

Acid and alkaline foods means how much acid or alkaline

the foods contain. Table 2 is a list of foods arranged by pH, a measurement of acidity. Smaller numbers mean stronger in acid, larger numbers mean weaker in acid. A pH of 7 is neutral and a pH larger than 7 is alkaline. This concept of acid and alkaline foods is commonly used. However, when nutritionists speak of acid or alkaline forming foods, that is different from the acid or alkaline foods listed in Table 2. They are talking about the acid forming ability or the alkaline forming ability of foods. In other words, limes, with a pH of 1.9, contain strong acid. However, they are an alkaline forming food. By acid forming or alkaline forming, nutritionists mean the condition foods cause in the body after being digested.

Most proteins in food combine with sulfur and many are also combined with phosphorus. When the protein is metabolized, these elements remain as sulfuric and phosphoric acid and must be neutralized by ammonia, calcium, sodium, and potassium before they can be excreted by the kidneys. This is the reason that high protein foods, especially animal foods, generally are acid forming foods. This is also true of most grains because they contain much sulfur and phosphorus.

In fruit and most vegetables, the organic acid (such as the acidity of an orange which you can taste) contains many elements such as potassium, sodium, calcium, and magnesium. Organic acids, when oxidized, become carbon dioxide and water; the alkaline elements (K, Na, Ca, Mg) remain and neutralize body acid. In other words, strangely enough, *acid foods reduce body acids.* This is the reason that fruits and most vegetables are considered alkaline forming foods. Conversely, high protein foods and most grains, when metabolized, produce acid that must be neutralized; therefore they are generally acid forming foods.

In short, there are two kinds of elements in our foods: acid forming elements and alkaline forming elements.

Acid forming elements	Alkaline forming elements
sulfur (S)	sodium (Na)
phosphorus (P)	potassium (K)
chlorine (Cl)	calcium (Ca)
iodine (I)	magnesium (Mg)
	iron (Fe)

Table 3. Average Amount of Minerals in a 154-lb. Adult Man

Acid forming elements		Alkaline forming elements	
Cl	85.000 gr.	Na	63 gr.
P	670.000 gr.	K	150 gr.
S	112.000 gr.	Ca	1,160 gr.
I	0.014 gr.	Mg	21 gr.
		Fe	3 gr.

Source: *Medical Physiology,* by Arthur Guyton, p. 858.

Table 4. Daily Requirement of Minerals for a 154-lb. Adult Man

Acid forming elements		Alkaline forming elements	
Cl	3.50000 gr.	Na	3.000 gr.
PO_4	1.50000 gr.	K	1.000 gr.
I	0.00025 gr.	Ca	0.800 gr.
		Mg	unknown
		Fe	0.012 gr.

Source: *Medical Physiology,* by Arthur Guyton, p. 858.

Calcium (alkaline forming element)

The Yearbook of Agriculture 1959, U. S. Department of Agriculture, states:

> Calcium, the most abundant mineral in the body, comprises 1.5 to 2.0 percent of the weight of an adult's body. It usually is associated with phosphorus. . . . [Phosphorus is an acid forming element.] A person who weighs 154 lbs. would have 2.3 to 3.1 lbs. of calcium and 1.2 to 1.7 lbs. of phosphorus in his body.
>
> About 99 percent of the calcium and 80 to 90 percent of the phosphorus are in the bones and teeth. The rest is in the soft tissues and body fluids and is highly important to their normal functioning.
>
> Calcium is essential for the clotting of blood, the action of certain enzymes, and the control of the passage of fluids through the cell walls. The right proportion of calcium in the blood is responsible for the alternate contraction and relaxation of the heart muscle.
>
> The irritability of the nerves is increased when the amount of calcium in the blood is below normal.
>
> Calcium in a complex combination with phosphorus gives rigidity and hardness to the bones and teeth. . . .
>
> The intricate process of bone building requires many nutrients besides calcium and phosphorus. Vitamin D is essential for absorption from the intestinal tract and the orderly deposition of the bone material. Protein is needed for the framework and for part of every cell and circulating fluid. Vitamin A aids in the deposition of the minerals. Vitamin C is required for the cementing material between the cells and the firmness of the walls of the blood vessels. . . .
>
> When there is no reserve to use, the calcium has to be taken from the bone structure itself – usually

first from the spine and pelvic bones. . . . If the calcium that is withdrawn in times of increased need is not replaced, the bone becomes deficient in calcium and subnormal in composition. From 10 to 40 percent of the normal amount of calcium may be withdrawn from mature bone before the deficiency will show on an X-ray film. . . .

The calcium that is absorbed travels in the blood to places where it is needed, particularly the bones. If any of the absorbed calcium is not needed, it is excreted by the kidneys into the urine. Normal functioning of the kidneys is essential for the normal metabolism of calcium and other minerals.

Vitamin D is essential for the absorption of calcium from the gastrointestinal tract. Vitamin D does not occur naturally in many foods. Egg yolk, butter, fortified margarine, and certain fish oils are the chief sources.

A special substance, ergosterol, is present in the skin and is changed to vitamin D by the ultraviolet rays of the sun.

In the macrobiotic diet, we don't eat much meat, chicken, or fish and we don't drink milk either. It seems to me that vitamin D is supplied sufficiently through sunshine. If children show a deficiency of calcium (such as rickets), milk, cod liver oil, or small fish (whole) are recommended. If you are afraid of a shortage of vitamin D, please eat mushrooms.

According to James Moon, 'vitamin D' is a hormone, derived from animal sources (see *Macrobiotic Explanation of Pathological Calcification*, by J. Moon). I speculate that we are able to produce enough vitamin D if we are on a balanced natural diet.

"The concentration of *calcium in the blood plasma* of most mammals and many vertebrates is remarkably constant at about 2.5 mM (10 mg./100 ml. of plasma). In the plasma,

Table 5. Vitamin D Content in Various Foods

Total International Units in 100 gr. of Food			
cow's milk	0.003	butter	0.1
human milk	0.002	mackerel	12.0
egg	0.070	cod fish	2.5
pork liver	0.010	shiitake mushroom	2639.0
beef liver	0.010	pine mushroom	2103.0
sardines	0.045	yeasted bread	3657.0

(Japanese National Nutrition Research Institute)

calcium exists in three forms: as the free ion, bound to proteins, and complexed with organic (*e.g.*, citrate) or inorganic (*e.g.*, phosphate) acids. The free ion accounts for about 47.5% of the plasma calcium; 46% is bound to proteins and 6.5% is in complexed form. Of the latter, phosphate and citrate account for half." (Williams and Lansford, *The Encyclopedia of Biochemistry*, p. 162.)

According to *The Yearbook of Agriculture 1959:*

> The parathyroid hormone keeps the amount of calcium in the blood at a normal level of about 10 milligrams per 100 milliliters of blood serum. (Serum is the watery part of the blood that separates from a clot.)
>
> Any wide deviation from this amount is dangerous to health and life. [Katase's opinion about this is in the latter part of this chapter.] The hormone can shift calcium and phosphorus from the bone into the blood. If the blood levels are too high, it can increase the excretion of these minerals by the kidneys. If anything reduces the secretion of the parathyroid hormone, the calcium in the blood drops quickly, the phosphorus rises, and severe muscular twitchings result.

Table 6. Ratio of Calcium/Phosphorus Content
in Various Foods (100 gr. samples)

Name	Ca (mg.)	P (mg.)	Ca/P	Name	Ca (mg.)	P (mg.)	Ca/P
hijiki	1400	56	25.1	chicken	4	280	0.01
radish leaves	190	30	6.3	pork	4	180	0.02
kombu	800	150	5.3	bonita	6	220	0.03
wakame	1300	260	5.0	tuna	11	350	0.03
bancha	720	200	3.6	white rice	6	170	0.04
nori	600	200	3.0	codfish	9	160	0.06
carrot leaves	200	74	2.7	mackerel	22	300	0.07
scallions (green)	100	51	2.0	bamboo shoots	4	51	0.08
spinach	98	52	2.0	salmon	22	240	0.09
sesame seeds (black)	1100	570	1.9	white bread	11	68	0.16
tofu	160	86	1.9	eggs	65	230	0.28
radishes	28	17	1.6	miso	81	180	0.45
tangerines	16	14	1.1	eggplant	16	26	0.62
milk	100	90	1.1	cucumbers	19	27	0.70
yoghurt	150	140	1.0	sweet potatoes	24	33	0.73
				Chinese cabbage	33	40	0.83
				carrots (root)	47	60	0.78
				scallions (white)	50	51	0.98

*(The bigger the Ca/P ratio, the more alkaline; the smaller the ratio, the
more acid. A more detailed treatment of much of this material can be found
in Table 10 on page 43.)*

Phosphorus (acid forming element)

Phosphorus is 0.8 to 1.1 percent of the body weight. Phosphorus is an essential part of every living cell. It takes part in the chemical reactions with proteins, fats, and carbohydrates to give the body energy and vital materials for growth and repair; for example, the phospholipids, which are important in the synthesis of cell membranes and synthesis of DNA and RNA. Phosphorus helps the blood neutralize acids and alkalies. Along with calcium, phosphorus works for the formation of bones and teeth.

Adults should have the same amount of phosphorus as they have calcium. Children should have about one and one-half times as much phosphorus as calcium. The needs of normal people for phosphorus are supplied by the same foods that supply their needs for calcium and protein, so diets that provide enough of these elements very likely furnish enough phosphorus as well.

Since phosphorus exists abundantly in animal foods, and phosphorus produces poisonous acid, the macrobiotic diet recommends less animal foods. Table 6 (p. 28) shows that animal foods contain too much phosphorus and that vegetables and seaweeds contain good proportions of calcium and phosphorus.

The name phosphorus came from the Greek *phosphoros* meaning light bearing, symbolized by P; a nonmetallic chemical element of the nitrogen family. It is a colorless, soft, waxy solid that glows in the dark. It has a great affinity with oxygen. It fires spontaneously upon exposure to air and forms dense white fumes of the oxide. It is essential to plant and animal life. Phosphorus was first prepared in elemental form in 1669 by a German alchemist, Henning Brand, from a residue of evaporated urine.

Phosphorus is present in the fluids within the cells of

living tissues as the phosphate ion, PO_4^-, one of the most important mineral constituents needed for cellular activity. The genes, which direct heredity and other cellular functions and are found in the nucleus of each cell, are molecules of DNA (deoxyribonucleic acid) which all contain phosphorus. Cells store the energy obtained from nutrients in molecules of adenosine triphosphate (ATP). Calcium phosphate is the principal inorganic constituent of teeth and bones.

Potassium and Sodium (alkaline forming elements)

A Japanese military doctor named Sagen Ishizuka reached the conclusion after 40 years of medical research that the amount of potassium and sodium in foods is the key factor which determines strength of body, adaptability to the weather, climatic influence over the character and mentality of man, growth characteristics of plants, etc., which I will discuss in the next chapter.

According to *The Yearbook of Agriculture 1959:*

> Sodium, potassium, and magnesium are essential in nutrition. They are among the most plentiful minerals in the body. Calcium and phosphorus are present in the largest amounts, and then come potassium, sulfur, sodium, chlorine, and magnesium in descending order of amounts.
>
> A person who weighs 154 pounds has about 9 ounces of potassium, and 4 ounces of sodium, and 1.3 ounces of magnesium in his body.
>
> Sodium and potassium are similar in chemical properties but different in their location within the body. Sodium is chiefly in the fluids that circulate outside the cells, and only a small amount of it is inside the cells. Potassium is mostly inside the cells, and a much smaller amount is in the body fluids.
>
> Sodium and potassium are vital in keeping a

normal balance of water between the cells and the fluids. A decline in the sodium content of the fluids results in a transfer of water from the fluids into the cells. An increase in sodium causes a transfer of water from the cells into the fluids.

Sodium and potassium are essential for nerves to respond to stimulation, for the nerve impulses to travel to the muscles, and for the muscles to contract. All types of muscles, including the heart muscle, are influenced by sodium and potassium.

Sodium and potassium also work with proteins, phosphates, and carbonates to keep a proper balance between the amount of acid and alkali in the blood.

One very interesting claim by Western science on K and Na can be found in the *Encyclopedia of Biochemistry* (p. 679):

> Sodium (Na) is essential to higher animals which regulate the composition of their body fluids and to some marine organisms, but it is dispensible for many bacteria and most plants, except for the blue-green algae. Potassium (K), on the other hand, is essential for all, or nearly all, forms of life. . . .
>
> Na and K are important constituents of both intra-and extracellular fluids. . . . Ringer found in 1882 that to maintain the contractillity of isolated frog heart, it was necessary to perfuse it with a medium containing Na, K and Ca ions in the proportion of seawater. It has since been recognized that the normal life activities of tissues and cells may depend on a proper balance among the inorganic cations to which they are exposed. Sodium is required for the sustained contractillity of mammalian muscle while K has a paralyzing effect; a balance is necessary for normal function.

Iron (alkaline forming element)

In *Medical Physiology*, Arthur Guyton states:

The major proportion of iron in the body is in the form of hemoglobin, though smaller quantities are present in other forms, especially in the liver and in the bone marrow. Electron carriers containing iron (especially the cytochromes) are present in all the cells of the body and are essential for most of the oxidation that occurs in the cells. Therefore, iron is absolutely essential both for transport of oxygen to the tissues, and for maintenance of oxidative systems within the tissue cells, without which life would cease within a few seconds.

Vegetables are a good source of iron, especially beefsteak leaves, which are used as coloring for umeboshi (salted dried plum). Meat, chicken, and fish have traces of iron, and cow's milk and human milk also have small amounts of iron.

Pregnant women must observe a diet which contains a good amount of iron, such as provided by miso soup.

Magnesium (alkaline forming element)

Magnesium is closely related to both calcium and phosphorus in its location and function in the body. About 70% of the magnesium in the body is in the bones. The rest is in the soft tissues and blood. Muscle tissue contains more magnesium than calcium. Blood contains more calcium than magnesium.

Magnesium acts as a starter or catalyzer for some of the chemical reactions within the body. It also becomes a part of some of the complex molecules that are formed as the body uses food for growth and for maintenance and repair. There is some relation between magnesium and the hormone cortisone, as they affect the amount of phosphate in the blood. Magnesium, primarily an intracellular ion, is distributed among all tissues. It constitutes about 0.05 percent of the animal body weight, and of this, 60 percent occurs in the skeleton and only 1 percent in the extracellular fluids. The rest is in the intracellular fluids.

According to Arthur Guyton, "Increased extracellular concentration of magnesium depresses activity in the nervous system and also depresses skeletal muscle contraction. This latter effect can be blocked by administration of calcium. Low magnesium concentration causes greatly increased irritability of the nervous system, peripheral vasodilatation, and cardiac arrhythmias."

Sulfur (acid forming element)

Sulfur is found in the elementary state mixed with earthy matter in volcanic districts, the chief supply being derived from Sicily. In *The Encyclopedia of Biochemistry*, Williams and Lansford state:

> Sulfur in some form is required by all living organisms. It is utilized in various oxidation states including sulfide, elemental sulfur, sulfite, sulfate and thiosulfate by lower forms, and in organic combination by all. The more important sulfur-containing organic compounds include: the amino acids, cysteine, cystine, and methonine which are components of protein; the vitamins thiamine and biotin; the cofactors, lipoic acid and co-enzyme A; certain complex lipids of nerve tissue, the sulfatides; . . . the hormones vasopressin and oxytocin; many therapeutic agents such as the sulfonamides and penicillins as well as most of the oral hypoglycemic agents used in the treatment of diabetes mellitus.

"In the organic world sulfur is built in the proteid molecules of the plant from the sulfates taken from the soil. It is chiefly taken up by the animal organism in the form of protein, and secreted for the most part in the highest oxidized condition as sulfuric acid, derived from the splitting up and oxidation of the protein molecule. In this form, combined and neutralized by alkalies, it is again ready to begin the cycle of life, by forming organic sulfur compounds in plants." (Carquel, *Vital Facts About Foods.)*

Chlorine (acid forming element)

Chlorine is found chiefly in sodium chloride or common salt, either dissolved in water or as solid deposit in the interior of the earth as rock salt. It is a poisonous gas.

Chlorine, in the form of sodium chloride, plays an important part in the animal organism. It assists in the formation of all the digestive juices, principally of the gastric juice, which contains two parts per 1 mille hydrochloric acid. The mineral matter of the blood serum is made up largely of sodium chloride, which favors and sustains the generation and conduction of electric currents. Chlorides are useful, not only in the construction of the organs but also in the preparation of the digestive secretions.

Chlorides are likewise important for anal secretion. They are necessary for the elimination of the nitrogenous waste products of metabolism.

CHAPTER III

Acid and Alkaline in Foods

1. Acid and Alkaline Forming Foods

All natural foods contain both acid and alkaline forming elements. In some, acid forming elements dominate; in others, alkaline forming elements dominate. According to modern biochemistry, it is not the organic matter of foods that leave acid or alkaline residues in the body. The inorganic matter (sulphur, phosphorus, potassium, sodium, magnesium and calcium) determines the acidity or alkalinity of the body fluids.

Foods comparatively rich in acid forming elements are acid forming foods; those comparatively rich in alkaline forming elements are alkaline forming foods:

Acid Forming Foods	Alkaline Forming Foods
eggs	salt
beef	miso
pork	soy sauce
chicken	vegetables
fish	fruits
cheese	wine
grains (most)	coffee
nuts, beans	
beer	
whiskey	
sugar	

2. How to Determine Acid Forming Foods and Alkaline Forming Foods

In theory, whether a given food is acid forming or alkaline forming is determined by the proportion of acid forming and alkaline forming elements contained in the food. In practical reality, however, it is determined by test tube. This procedure is known as titration.

First, the food to be measured is burned to ashes. (It is this step of burning the food that takes the place of digestion and thus gives us a picture of whether the food is acid or alkaline forming.) Next, a standard amount of very pure water, say one liter, is added to 100 grams of these ashes to make a solution. This solution is tested to see whether it is acid or alkaline. Once we know whether the solution is acid or alkaline, we can measure the concentration or strength of the acidity or alkalinity of the ash solution.

Since an acid solution will neutralize or cancel an alkaline solution, and vice versa, the two can be used to measure each other. Suppose that the ash of a given food produces an acid solution when it is mixed with pure water. We know that the solution is acidic, but the strength of this acid is still unknown to us. In order to determine the strength of the acidity of an unknown solution, an alkaline solution of known strength is added to the unknown acid until the two cancel each other and the solution reaches neutral.

As we go we keep track of how many milliliters of the known alkaline solution we add. The amount of alkaline solution required to neutralize the unknown acid is thus a good measure of the acidity of the original ash and water solution, and therefore of the acid forming strength of the food from which the ash solution was made.

In the same way, by noting how ma
acid solution of known strength it tak
unknown alkaline solution, we can mea
of an unknown alkaline ash and thus th
strength of the food from which the as

The following table presents an orde.ing of acid and
alkaline forming foods determined by the method described above (from the work of Dr. Hirotaro Nishizaki).
Under each heading the foods are listed from strongest to
weakest. The number which appears after each food in
the table tells how many milliliters of known solution
were required to neutralize the original ash solution.
These numbers give us a picture of the relative strengths
of the various acid and alkaline forming foods.

For instance, from Table 7 we learn that rice bran, the
most acid forming of the foods tested, is about 2.3 times
more acid forming than are bonita flakes, about 8.6 times
more acid forming than barley, and 852 times more acid
forming than asparagus.

On the alkaline side of the table we find that wakame is
about 4.6 times more alkaline forming than konnyaku,
about 25.6 times more alkaline forming than soybeans,
and 2608 times more alkaline forming than tofu.

Comparing the two sides of the table we also notice
interesting relations. Peanuts (acid forming) and potatoes
(alkaline forming) are about equally matched at 5.4 each.
The same is true of asparagus and tofu (0.1 each), carp and
banana (8.8 each), and oatmeal and shiitake (17.8 to 17.5).
On the other hand, scallop (6.6) is about twice as acid
forming as apples (3.4) are alkaline, pork (6.2) is thirty-
one times as acid forming as cow's milk (0.2) is alkaline,
and carrots (6.4) are twice as alkaline forming as shrimp
(3.2) is acid.

Table 7. Acid and Alkaline Forming Foods

Acid Forming Foods		Alkaline Forming Foods	
rice bran	85.2	wakame	260.8
bonita flakes	37.1	konnyaku	56.2
bream eggs	29.8	kombu	40.0
dried squid	29.6	ginger	21.1
dried fish	24.0	kidney beans	18.8
egg yolk	19.2	shiitake	17.5
oatmeal	17.8	spinach	15.6
brown rice	15.5	soybeans	10.2
tuna	15.3	bananas	8.8
octopus	12.8	chestnuts	8.3
sake no kasu	12.1	albi (taro)	7.7
chicken	10.4	azuki beans	7.3
pearled barley	9.9	carrots	6.4
carp	8.8	komatsuna	6.4
bream	8.6	mushrooms	6.4
oysters	8.0	kyona	6.2
salmon	7.9	strawberries	5.6
buckwheat flour	7.7	potatoes	5.4
eel	7.5	burdock	5.1
clam	7.5	radish pickles	5.0
horse meat	6.6	cabbage	4.9
scallops	6.6	radishes	4.6
pork	6.2	squash	4.4
peanuts	5.4	bamboo shoots	4.3
herring eggs	5.4	sweet potatoes	4.3
beef	5.0	turnips	4.2
fava beans	4.4	lotus root	3.8
cheese	4.3	orange juice	3.6
abalone	3.6	apples	3.4
whole barley	3.5	egg white	3.2

Table 7. continued

Acid Forming Foods		Alkaline Forming Foods	
shrimp	3.2	persimmons	2.7
peas	2.5	pears	2.6
beer	1.1	grape juice	2.3
bread	0.6	cucumbers	2.2
chicken soup	0.6	watermelon	2.1
age (fried tofu)	0.5	eggplant	1.9
sake (rice wine)	0.5	coffee	1.9
butter	0.4	onions	1.7
asparagus	0.1	tea	1.6
		bracken	1.6
		pickles (leaves)	1.3
		string beans	1.1
		human milk	0.5
		cow's milk	0.2
		tofu	0.1

Comments on Tables

Tables 7, 8, and 9 are translated from the Japanese book, *The Usefulness of Alkaline Forming Foods,* from the Women's University on Nutrition. Tables 8 and 9 contain the same data as Table 7, but classified in addition by the kinds of food. It is very interesting to find that rice bran is the most acid forming food while wakame is the most alkaline forming food. According to the list, butter is a weak acid forming food; however, because of its fat content, butter is really a stronger acid forming food than this method

Table 8. Acid Forming Foods

Animal	Grains	Beans	Other	Acidity
	rice bran			85.2
bonita flakes				37.1
bream eggs				29.8
dried squid				29.6
dried fish				24.0
egg yolk				19.2
	oatmeal			17.8
	brown rice			15.5
tuna				15.3
octopus				12.8
			sake no kasu	12.1
chicken				10.4
	pearled barley			9.9
carp				8.8
bream				8.6
oysters				8.0
salmon				7.9
	buckwheat flour			7.7
eel				7.5
clam				7.5
horse meat				6.6
scallops				6.6
pork				6.2
		peanuts		5.4
herring eggs				5.4
beef				5.0
		fava beans		4.4
cheese				4.3
	white rice			4.3
abalone				3.6
	whole barley			3.5
shrimp				3.2
	wheat gluten			3.0
		peas		2.5
			beer	1.1
	bread			0.6
			age	0.5
			sake	0.5
butter				0.4
			asparagus	0.1

Table 9. Alkaline Forming Foods

Vegetables	Fruits	Nuts/Beans	Other	Alkalinity
wakame				260.8
konnyaku				56.2
kombu				40.0
ginger				21.1
		kidney beans		18.8
shiitake				17.5
spinach				15.6
		soybeans		10.2
	bananas			8.8
		chestnuts		8.3
albi				7.7
		azuki beans		7.3
carrots				6.4
mushrooms				6.4
	strawberries			5.6
potatoes				5.4
burdock				5.1
radish pickles				5.0
cabbage				4.9
radishes				4.6
squash				4.4
bamboo shoots				4.3
sweet potatoes				4.3
lotus root				3.8
	orange juice			3.6
	apples			3.4
			egg white	3.2
	persimmons			2.7
	pears			2.6
	grape juice			2.3
cucumbers				2.2
	watermelon			2.1
eggplant				1.9
			coffee	1.9
onions				1.7
bracken				1.6
			tea	1.6
		string beans		1.1
			human milk	0.5
			cow's milk	0.2
		tofu		0.1

indicates. This method is not suitable to measure acidity and alkalinity of some foods such as butter and beans which are high in fat. These foods should be placed higher on the list of acid forming foods than they are here.

If we cannot find measurements of the acid or alkaline forming character of a food that we are interested in, we can still determine these properties approximately by using the ratio of calcium and phosphorus content of the food in question. The disadvantage of this method is that it works better for making an approximation of acid forming foods than for alkaline forming foods, and I will say more about this below. The advantage of this approach is that information on the amount of calcium and phosphorus present in foods can be found in most food composition books.

For our purposes, calcium represents the alkaline forming elements in food, and phorphorus represents the acid forming elements. The following table shows acid and alkaline forming characteristics of various foods based on the ratio of their calcium and phosphorus content as follows:

Ca/P Ratio	Result
greater than 3.00	strong alkaline forming
2.99 to 2.00	alkaline forming
1.99 to 1.00	weak alkaline forming
0.99 to 0.50	weak acid forming
0.49 to 0.20	acid forming
less than 0.20	strong acid forming

The values for calcium (Ca) and phosphorus (P) listed in Table 10 are taken from *Composition of Foods*, published by the United States Department of Agriculture.

Table 10. The Calcium and Phosphorus Ratio: Ca/P

Foods	Calcium	Phosphorus	Ca/P
Animal, Fish & Shell Fish			
alkaline forming			
human milk	33	14	2.36
weak alkaline forming			
cheese, cheddar	750	478	1.57
cow's milk	118	93	1.27
goat's milk	129	106	1.22
yoghurt, whole	111	97	1.14
weak acid forming			
cheese, American	697	771	0.90
caviar	276	355	0.77
oyster, raw	94	143	0.66
cheese, cottage	94	152	0.62
egg white	9	15	0.60
acid forming			
salmon	79	186	0.42
shrimp, raw	63	166	0.38
egg, whole	54	205	0.26
crab, cooked	43	175	0.25
egg yolk	141	569	0.25
strong acid forming			
abalone	37	191	0.19
carp	50	253	0.19
scallops, raw	26	208	0.13
bacon	13	108	0.12
cod, raw	10	104	0.10
flounder	23	344	0.07
pork, raw	5	88	0.06
beef, T-Bone steak	8	135	0.06
halibut, raw	13	211	0.06
ham	9	170	0.05
chicken, skinned	11	265	0.04
turkey, skinned	8	212	0.04
mackerel, raw	8	274	0.03

Table 10. continued

Foods	Calcium	Phosphorus	Ca/P
Grain			
acid forming			
buckwheat, groats	114	282	0.40
bread, whole wheat	90	228	0.39
rice, long grain	60	200	0.30
rice, white	24	94	0.26
strong acid forming			
rice, brown	32	221	0.14
wheat, winter	46	354	0.13
oats, raw	70	590	0.12
rye, whole	38	378	0.10
wheat, whole, red	36	383	0.09
barley, pearled	16	189	0.08
corn meal	20	256	0.08
millet	20	311	0.06
corn, sweet, raw	3	111	0.03
Beans & Nuts			
acid forming			
beans, lima	52	142	0.37
chestnuts, fresh	27	88	0.31
soybeans	67	225	0.30
beans, red	110	406	0.27
walnuts, English	99	380	0.26
lentils, raw	79	377	0.21
strong acid forming			
peanuts, raw	69	401	0.17
coconuts	13	95	0.14
cashews	38	373	0.10
Other Acid Forming Foods			
weak acid forming			
baking powder	1923	2904	0.66
honey	5	6	0.83
soy milk	30	59	0.51

Table 10. continued

Foods	Calcium	Phosphorus	Ca/P
Vegetables & Sea Vegetables			
strong alkaline forming			
Irish moss, raw	885	157	5.64
rhubarb, raw	96	18	5.33
kelp, raw	1093	240	4.55
mustard greens	183	50	3.66
parsley, raw	203	63	3.22
spinach, raw	93	31	3.00
alkaline forming			
kale, raw	249	93	2.68
weak alkaline forming			
cabbage, raw	49	29	1.69
endive	81	54	1.50
celery, raw	39	28	1.39
lettuce, raw	35	26	1.35
radishes, daikon	35	26	1.35
broccoli, raw	103	78	1.32
turnips, raw	39	30	1.30
pickles, dill	26	21	1.24
dulse, raw	296	267	1.11
cabbage, Chinese	43	40	1.07
carrots, raw	37	36	1.03
weak acid forming			
Swiss chard, raw	38	39	0.97
summer squash	28	29	0.96
zucchini	28	29	0.96
cucumbers, raw	25	27	0.93
onions, raw	27	36	0.75
parsnips, raw	50	77	0.65
ginger, fresh	23	36	0.64
acid forming			
pumpkin, raw	21	44	0.48
tomatoes, ripe	13	27	0.48
eggplant, raw	12	26	0.46
taro, raw	28	61	0.46
cauliflower, raw	25	56	0.44
asparagus, raw	22	62	0.35
avocados, raw	10	42	0.23

Table 10. continued

Foods	Calcium	Phosphorus	Ca/P
strong acid forming			
garlic, raw	29	202	0.14
potatoes, raw	7	53	0.13
mushrooms, raw	6	116	0.05
yeast, dry	44	1291	0.03
Fruits & Seeds			
strong alkaline forming			
maple sugar	143	11	13.00
brown sugar	85	19	4.47
alkaline forming			
tangerines	40	18	2.20
oranges, raw	41	20	2.00
weak alkaline forming			
sesame seeds	1160	616	1.88
lemons, raw	26	16	1.63
grapefruit	32	20	1.60
figs, raw	35	22	1.59
currants, raw	60	40	1.50
grapes, raw	16	12	1.33
cherries, raw	22	19	1.16
blueberries, raw	10	9	1.10
plums, raw	18	17	1.06
strawberries	21	21	1.00
weak acid forming			
dates	59	63	0.94
wine	9	10	0.90
apricots	17	23	0.73
apples	7	10	0.70
raisins, raw	62	101	0.61
acid forming			
bananas, raw	8	26	0.30
chocolate	78	384	0.20
strong acid forming			
sunflower seeds	120	837	0.14

As I mentioned above, determining the acid and alkaline forming character of foods by using their calcium/phosphorus ratio is convenient. It is not always accurate, however. Millet is a food where this inaccuracy is most obvious. Millet is generally thought to be an alkaline forming grain, but from its Ca/P ratio it is grouped with the acid forming foods. Considering the differences between the two methods of determining which foods are acid forming and which are alkaline forming, Tables 19 and 20 are offered to correct Table 10.

3. Fat and Acid Alkaline Balance

Fat is considered one of the three major nutrients: namely carbohydrates, proteins, and fats. From the viewpoint of the natural food diet, fat has been given too much importance. Fat is, however, a source of linoleic acid and vitamins A and D. If animals are fed without fat, they will eventually die. However, if these animals are fed with a little amount of linoleic acid, they grow without trouble. In other words, the linoleic acid contained in fat is important. Since linoleic acid is contained in rice as well as in soy beans, we don't worry about its lack as long as we follow a basic diet of whole grains and vegetables, such as the macrobiotic natural food diet.

There are two kinds of fat: animal fat and vegetal fat. Both contain poisonous compounds; however, animal fat is more poisonous. Even cod liver oil causes acidosis if it is consumed too much. According to Dr. Katase in *Calcium Medicine*:

> A 110 lb. adult achieved the best result (alkaline condition of blood) when he consumed only $1/_5$ oz. of cod liver oil. This same person had an apparent acidosis when he consumed 1 oz. of the oil. . . . Milk

fat, that is to say butter, is commonly considered the best fat among the foods. Butter contains calcium and vitamins. However, giving more than 4 oz. of butter to a person weighing 110 lbs. caused acidosis and lack of calcium. . . . Fats easier to melt cause a more acidic condition than harder ones. The cause of baldness is too much consumption of fat.

4. Carbohydrates and Acid Alkaline Balance

Carbohydrates are the source of our energy. A carbohydrate consists of carbon, hydrogen, and oxygen. The formula of any of these compounds may be expressed as $C_m(H_2O)_n$.

There are three types of carbohydrates. The simplest carbohydrates are the monosaccharides, of which the most important for us is glucose. Next are the disaccharides, which are made by two monosaccharide molecules joined together by an oxygen atom, with the elimination of a molecule of water. The most important disaccharides are sucrose (ordinary cane sugar), lactose, and maltose. The third type of carbohydrates are the polysaccharides, which have enormous molecules made of many monosaccharide units – about 10 for glycogen, 25 for starch, and 100 to 200 for cellulose.

Having small molecules, monosaccharides reach the intestinal wall and are absorbed directly into the body without any change of chemical compounds. Since disaccharides have slightly larger molecules, they must be broken down to monosaccharides by various enzymes. That is to say, sucrose will be broken down to glucose by invertase, maltose by maltase, and lactose by lactase. Then this simple sugar is absorbed through the intestinal wall. The absorption of monosaccharides and disaccharides is very fast, and within a short time digested glucose enters into the bloodstream. This upsets the glucose balance in the blood. However, the case of polysaccharides is different. Having large molecules, polysaccharides (such as glycogen, starch and cellulose) have to pass many digestive processes. At first, those carbohydrates are broken down to the disaccharides (sucrose, maltose and lactose) by the action of the enzyme called amirose. Then those disaccharides are broken down to monosaccharides, such as glucose, by the action of their own enzymes. The final monosaccharides (glucose) will be absorbed into the bloodstream as they are made. In other words, monosaccharides produced from polysaccharides will be absorbed much later and slower than mono or disaccharides. Therefore, glucose produced from polysaccharides such as grains will never upset the glucose balance of the bloodstream. Since monosaccharides and disaccharides are absorbed quickly, the amount of glucose in the body cells increases. The result is an imbalance of oxygen, causing incomplete burning. This incomplete burning produces many organic acids such as lactic acid, pyro-racemic acid, butyric acid, and acetic acid. This is an example of acidosis or an acidic condition caused by the overeating of candy or fruits. (Source of information: Katase, *Calcium Medicine*.)

5. Sugar and Acid Alkaline Balance

For the reason mentioned above, sugar has a tendency to cause an acidic condition. Black sugar is less acid forming, however, because it is a less processed sugar. It contains alkaline forming minerals and vitamins which help the combustion of glucose in the body.

According to Dr. T. Katase, "The minimum amount of

sugar to cause an acidic condition in 5 to 6 year old children is 1/5 oz. for 40 lbs. weight, 1/4 oz. for 50 lbs. weight, and 3/10 oz. for 60 lbs. weight. It is important for the health of children to make a character of disliking sugar and sugary foods. In order to build such a character in children, never give your baby sugar and sugary products after weaning. Instead, give dry kombu or daikon pickles. Such babies will dislike sugary foods after they grow up."

However, if children unfortunately have a habit of eating sugary foods already, the macrobiotic principle advises the following foods and activities:

1. Main foods should consist of grains, cereals, and bread.
2. Secondary foods should consist of seasonal vegetables and sea vegetables.
3. If you give any fruit, let them eat the skin also.
4. Don't give any refined, chemicalized, or processed foods.
5. Be active by playing outdoors always.
6. Don't wear warm clothes. Let them feel cold or cool in winter, hot in summer. Also, be a little hungry all the time.

This is the best way to maintain the body fluid alkaline, and the metabolism most functional. The following books are recommended by this author:

Sugar Blues – William Dufty
Sugar, Curse of Civilization – J. I. Rodale
Degeneration – Regeneration – Melvin Page
Nutrition and Physical Degeneration – Weston A. Price, D.D.S.
Sweet and Dangerous – John Yudkin, M.D.

6. Vitamins and Acid Alkaline Balance

Lack of vitamin A causes eye trouble; lack of vitamin B causes beriberi; lack of vitamin C causes scurvy; and lack of vitamin D causes rickets.

Dr. T. Katase experimented on the relationship between the acid alkaline balance and vitamins, using animals. As a result, he found these interesting relationships: vitamin B is a useful factor in maintaining the acid alkaline balance in the case of overeating protein; vitamin A is a useful factor in the case of overeating fat; vitamin C is a useful factor in the case of overeating carbohydrates and sugar; and vitamin D relates to all of them.

If vitamins are taken too much in pill form, they may cause acidosis. Vitamins from natural foods do not usually cause acidosis.

Vitamin A is contained in the following foods: liver of cow or pig, egg yolk, cheese, squash, shiso (beefsteak leaves), celery, radish leaves, red pepper leaves, carrot, carrot leaves, scallion, parsley, green pepper, mugwort, nori, hijiki, wakame (sea vegetables), Japanese tea, etc.

Vitamin B is contained in the following foods: brown rice, barley, mochi (sweet rice), wheat, walnuts, sesame seeds, azuki beans (red beans), cabbage, Japanese tea, burdock, etc.

Vitamin C is contained well in the following foods: citrus fruits, red pepper, carrot leaves, parsley, spinach, persimmon leaves, Japanese tea, etc.

Vitamin D is contained in animal fat as is ergosterol, which changes to vitamin C by ultraviolet light. Vitamin D is contained in the following foods in large amounts: shiitake (Japanese) mushrooms, mushrooms, yeast, cod liver oil, and any fish liver oil.

Dr. Katase recommended fruits, radish juice, orange

juice, etc., to alkalize acid caused by sugar. This is true in
the acid and alkaline balance only. However, from the
macrobiotic point of view, those foods are all very yin and
sugar is yin. Therefore, this type of diet will cause a very
yin condition, even though acid and alkaline may be balanced. I will explain this more in the next chapter.

"A Danish investigator, Carl Peter Henrik Dam, isolated a fat-soluble substance from dried alfalfa leaves.
Because it corrected the clotting or coagulating time of
the blood, he called it the Koagulations Vitamin. This was
shortened to vitamin K for convenience." (*The Yearbook of
Agriculture 1959.*) Vitamin K is not only effective for causing coagulation, but also for causing urination, detoxica-
tion, and antibacterial function. A Japanese doctor and
professor of physiology at Kyushu University, Dr. Goto,
applied vitamin K in the treatment of tuberculosis, gall
bladder infection, high blood pressure, liver infection, and
cancer with good results. However, nobody could explain
why vitamin K was effective for those diseases. It is Dr. F.
Yanagisawa who explained the function of vitamin K in
our body. He examined the calcium ion in human and
animal blood serum, giving vitamin K. The result was
amazing. Vitamin K increases the number of Ca ions in
the blood serum.

Seventy percent of our body weight is liquid, which is
distributed inside the cells, blood, and among tissues in
the following proportions:

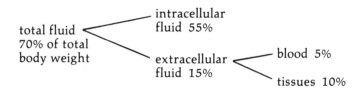

According to Dr. Yanagisawa in *Wheat for Health*, calcium exists only in the extracellular fluids, of which one-third is blood serum and two-thirds is tissue fluids. In this serum there are 10 mg. of calcium to every 100 ml. of serum, in the healthy condition. This 10 mg. of calcium consists of two kinds of calcium: 6 mg. are calcium protein compounds, and 4 mg. are ionized calcium. In a healthy person, the ratio of calcium compounds and calcium ions is 6:4, as mentioned above. However, when one becomes sick or tired, the number of calcium ions diminishes to a lower amount. When it reaches 1.5 mg. per 100 ml. of serum, one dies.

The decreased number of calcium ions is the result of increased numbers of calcium protein (globline) compounds. In other words, the increase of calcium globlines means the decrease of calcium ions. Calcium ions also have the same reverse relationship with phosphorus ions. When the number of calcium ions decreases, the number of phosphorus ions increases, and vice versa. Since calcium is an alkaline forming element and phosphorus is acid forming, the increased number of calcium ions causes an alkaline condition in the body fluids.

Dr. Yanagisawa examined the calcium ions of a seaman who was suffering from atomic radiation received from the Bikini Atomic Bomb Test. Dr. Yanagisawa confirmed the relationship between the number of Ca ions and sicknesses, and he could even predict the seaman's death by counting the calcium ions.

In short, about 40 percent of calcium in the blood serum must be ionized. Less than 40 percent means that one is in the beginning stages of disease. Dr. Yanagisawa concluded that vitamin K will ionize calcium. He produced and sold pills made of vitamin K taken from a wild grass. He made a lot of money. Dr. H. Goto recommended vitamin K for the treatment of tuberculosis. In both cases vitamin K helps to ionize calcium, because without ionization calcium is useless in our body.

Both doctors used vitamin K as a medicine and earned money. We don't need such a medicine, however, because vitamin K is abundant in nature. Vitamin K exists in green vegetables, especially in the outside leaves of cabbage. Pine leaves and bamboo leaves also contain vitamin K. According to Arthur Guyton, "Because vitamin K is synthesized by bacteria in the colon, a dietary source for this vitamin is not usually necessary, but when the bacteria of the colon are destroyed by administration of large quantities of antibiotic drugs, vitamin K deficiency occurs readily because of the paucity of this compound in the normal diet." (Guyton, *Medical Physiology*, p. 858.)

7. Conclusion

In *Calcium Medicine*, Dr. Katase states:

> In the intercellular fluid, there are four kinds of alkaline elements, Na, K, Ca, and Mg, in ionic condition. Also, there exist all nutrients delivered by blood, hormones, and waste products of metabolism. Those nutrients must enter the inside of the cell, passing through cell membranes in order to be utilized by the cells. This passing ability is dependent on the quantity and proportion of the ionic condition of the four alkaline elements. This is the osmotic pressure of cell membranes.
>
> In other words, when the four alkaline elements are the proper quantity, with the proper proprotions, the cells absorb the highest amount of nutrients and thus will be in the most healthy condition. At that time, we are the most healthy. If cells are sick, we are sick. Therefore, the condition of our health is dependent upon the condition of alkaline elements in the body fluids.

The four alkaline elements keep the blood or inter-cellular fluid alkaline, even though the body metabolism produces lots of acid. However, cell vitality and resistance to bacteria are further increased when alkalinity is a-chieved by Ca and/or Na, rather than K and/or Mg.

Dr. Katase cultured tuberculosis bacteria using these minerals. Ca and Na stopped the growth of the bacteria, but K and Mg increased the growth of the bacteria. Dr. Katase couldn't discover the reason for this. In order to clarify this phenomenon, I will explain the differences of Na and K in the next chapter.

The following chart has been added to verify how alka-line forming elements (Na, K, Ca, Mg) are balanced with acid forming elements (Cl, S, P) in our body fluids.

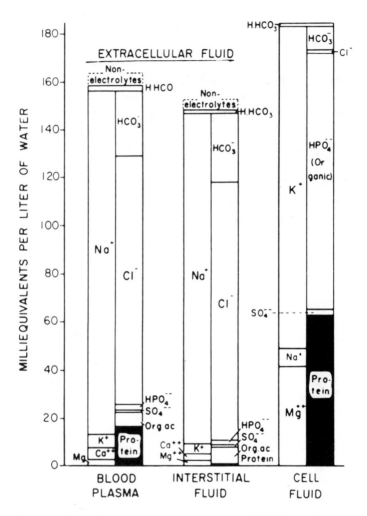

The composition of plasma, interstitial fluid, and intracellular fluid. (From Guyton, *Medical Physiology*.)

CHAPTER IV

Yin and Yang –
The Eastern Approach

1. Dr. Sagen Ishizuka – Founder of Japanese Macrobiotic Medicine and Diet

Sagen Ishizuka was born on February 4, 1851 at Fukui prefecture, two years before Admiral Perry arrived at Uraga Port asking to open trade between Japan and America.

He liked to study ever since he was young. He could understand Dutch, French, German, and English at age eighteen. Furthermore, his purpose in studying languages was not merely for the languages themselves. He studied in order to understand chemistry, medicine, and astronomy in those languages.

He had a skin disease by birth. When he was four, he suffered from prurigo over his whole body, and at five he suffered from acute kidney disease. This kidney disease was the cause of his death at age fifty-nine. His skin disease was caused by the kidney disease, which in turn was caused by his mother who ate too much fish and spices during her pregnancy. This he learned later, through macrobiotic medicine and diet. He established a unique medicine from his studies of Oriental medicine.

He suffered from this skin disease (kidney disease) during his lifetime. At twenty-eight, while he was on duty as an army doctor at Seinan Senso (the riot caused by T. Saigo, the famous army general of Kagoshima), the disease caused severe swelling in his legs and eyelids, and protein secretions in the urine. At the age of thirty-two, he suffered from the severe kidney disease again. At that time he started to study the relationship of food to sickness (macrobiotic medicine and nutrition).

He tried to cure his sickness through Western medicine at first, or rather we can say that he was interested in studying medicine because of his desire to cure his chronic disease. After finding that Western medicine didn't make him any better, he started to study Oriental medicine. After studying both medicines, he finally found right foods to bring health to the Japanese. The *Nei Ching* says, "There are three categories of drugs; the lowest one of which is poisonous, the second one is a little poisonous, the highest one is no poison. The lowest drug cures six out of ten sicknesses, leaving poisons in the patients. The middle one cures seven out of ten sicknesses, leaving a small amount of poison. Even the highest medicine can cure only eight or nine out of ten sicknesses. The sicknesses that medicine cannot cure can be cured only by foods."

Sagen reached the conclusion that foods are the highest medicine, after searching Western medicine for many years. He realized that all sickness and physical weakness is caused by wrong eating habits. In other words, he established a science of Foods for Health and Happiness. This is called *shokuyo* in Japanese, and was later called *macrobiotics* by George Ohsawa.

What is shokuyo? *Shoku* is all matter and energy which creates and nourishes the perfect man. *Yo* is the deed or way to nourish ourselves, with the knowledge of *shoku*. In other words, *shokuyo* is the right knowledge and proper deeds concerning creation and nourishment of the perfectly healthy man.

The spirit or attitude of *shokuyo* medicine, which he applied to the sick, was entirely opposite that of Western medicine. He advised an azuki bean, brown rice diet for stomach disease, which a Western medical doctor would not dare to advise due to the belief that brown rice is hard to digest. He also advised burdock root, radish juice, brown rice, etc., in which there are no therapeutic value in modernized Japanese thought. He emphasized improved physical resistance against diseases, rather than curing sicknesses symptomatically.

Finally he reached the idea which divides all foods into two categories. One is the potassium category and the other is the sodium category. He explained not only sicknesses but also natural phenomena, such as seasonal changes and differentiation of living things, by potassium and sodium.

At the time of Ishizuka, nutritional theory was interested mostly in the three organic nutrients: namely, protein, fat, and carbohydrate. In his opinion, the organic nutrients will compose most of the body; however, the inorganic minerals will control the functioning of the organs, the metabolism, and the activities of the nervous system. According to Ishizuka, the most important inorganic minerals in our body are potassium (K) and sodium (Na). These two minerals have very similar characteristics, and it is difficult to distinguish one from the other. However, when they combine with acid and form salts, those salts are quite distinguishable. Potassium salts and sodium salts are antagonistic to each other in their function in the body – like the wife and husband in a family. Not only are they opposed to each other, they are complementary – as a wife relies on her husband and a husband relies on his wife. If we compare nutrients to the army, he said, carbohydrates are the soldiers which make up the majority of the army; proteins and fats are the officers; potassium is a general, while sodium is a lieutenant general.

Potassium salt activates oxidation and sodium salt inhibits oxidation. To illustrate this: add ash paste to a string and dry well. Tie a safety pin or paper clip to one end of the string, and hang the other end somewhere it can hang freely. Then burn the string. The pin will fall down as the string burns. Next, add salt (NaCl) to a piece of string and dry it well. Follow the same procedure, hanging the string with the pin somewhere freely, and burn it. The string will burn up, but black ashes will keep the pin from falling, because the salt on the string prevents complete oxidation. The incomplete combustion makes black ashes.

Therefore, if one eats grains and vegetables, which contain much potassium, the blood will oxidize well and allow better physiological functioning. On the other hand, if one eats a lot of meats, poultry, fish, and eggs, which contain high amounts of sodium, blood oxidation is not so good, and leaves much poisonous acid. Therefore, vegetarians live longer and eaters of animal food live a shorter life. Since the air near the ocean has more sodium than the air in the mountains, people who live near the ocean have shorter lives than people who live in the mountains.

K salt catches fire and burns quickly, but also has the characteristic of reducing heat and keeping cool. Contrary to K salt, Na salt burns slower, and has the characteristic of increasing heat and keeping warm. For example, firewood grown far from the ocean catches fire easily and burns well; the ashes are white. K salt has been used in medicine for heat reduction. If one applies ash paste over the skin, it keeps the skin cool. In contrast, it is more difficult to start a fire with firewood grown at the ocean-side, and the wood burns more slowly. The ashes are black.

The Japanese custom is to cremate a person who dies. If he has been vegetarian the ash will be white, but if he has been eating a lot of animal foods the ash will be black. Therefore, if a monk dies and his ash is black, he proves himself to have been not a very highly spiritual monk. If his ash is white, he is proven to have been a spiritual, honest monk.

Dr. Ishizuka discusses K salt and Na salt much more in his *Chemical Diet for Longevity*. He claims that physiological differences (such as color of the skin, fat or thin, big or small, speed of growth, strength, longevity, sickness, voice, good or bad memory, etc.) are all dependent on environmental conditions and the intake of K salt and Na salt foods. Dr. Ishizuka applied this K salt and Na salt relationship to his patients. He advised eating more K salt type foods if the symptoms are Na type. If the patient has a K salt type sickness, he advised eating Na type foods.

After his book was published, he was so famous that he had to consult one hundred patients every day. His treatment used no medicines, but dietary suggestions exclusively. People thought the diet he recommended was out-dated. However, his advice cured so many people that he became more and more famous. Letters from patients could reach him addressed merely: "Tokyo, Dr. Anti-Doctor."

After his death, his disciples established the *Shokuyo Kai Macrobiotic Association*. When this association was almost bankrupt, a young man who had cured his many sick-nesses by the brown rice diet of Dr. Ishizuka worked hard, putting his money to reorganize the Association. The Association became famous again and hundreds of patients came every day. This young man was George Ohsawa. He was not only good at business, but he also studied hard on Ishizuka's theory.

When Ohsawa learned Ishizuka's theory, he realized that a concept which explained the relationship between the two salts of K and Na had existed in the Orient for thousands of years. After several years of study, he changed Ishizuka's K salt and Na salt to the terminology of yin and yang.

2. George Ohsawa – Founder of Present-Day Macrobiotics

George Ohsawa (Nyoichi Sakurazawa) was born on October 18, 1893 in Kyoto, Japan. His mother and father had just moved to Kyoto from their locality to find a job. He said that his mother delivered him at the front of the *Tenryu-ji* temple. Therefore, there is a macrobiotic restaurant in Paris called *Tenryu* in honor of this episode.

Ohsawa was elected editor and manager of *Shokuyo Kai*. He was very busy with consultations, writing, and lectures. Ohsawa published probably his first macrobiotic diet and medicine book, *Lecture Series on Shokuyo*, in 1928. In this book, Ohsawa discusses the more spiritual side of diet; however, the basic theory is the same as Dr. Ishizuka's, except for one thing. Ohsawa called acid yang and alkaline yin. This was probably because acid changes blue litmus paper red, and alkaline changes red litmus paper blue – red being yang and blue being yin.

Later, when he lectured on macrobiotics for the first time in New York in January of 1960, he claimed acid is yin and alkaline yang. Since he classified grain as a yang food, many macrobiotic students had the idea that grains are alkaline. They were surprised when they learned that most grains are acid forming. When Ohsawa claimed that acid is yin and grains are yang, he was not discussing them on the same level. The statement "acid is yin" means that acid, compared with alkaline, is more yin. The statement "grains are yang" means that grains are yang when they are compared with vegetables. Secondly, Ohsawa didn't clarify the difference between acid or alkaline food and acid or alkaline *forming* foods, as I have already discussed in the previous chapters.

In my opinion, there are yin and yang in the acid forming foods as well as in the alkaline forming foods. This will be discussed in the next chapter. However, before doing so, I must give you more information on yin and yang.

3. Yin and Yang

The concept of yin and yang existed not only in the Orient, it existed in all of the ancient world. According to Greek mythology, there were Chaos and Earth at the beginning. From Chaos came Erebus and Night; from Night, the Ether (upper air) and Day. Earth (solid) first produced the Sea (liquid; the Ocean). (From Pinsent, *Greek Mythology.*)

According to Indian mythology, Shiva is the destroyer and Vishnu is the preserver. "With this eye he kills all the gods and other creatures during the periodic destructions of the Universe." (Ions, *Indian Mythology.*) In the same book: "As the preserver he is the embodiment of the quality of mercy and goodness, the self-existent, all-pervading power which preserves and maintains the universe and the cosmic order, dharma."

Thus Shiva represents the male power of the Universe,

and Vishnu the female power. In the *I Ching* (Book of Changes), *chien* represents the strong power, father and heaven, and *kien* is the yielding, mother and earth. In ancient China, strength, violence, blight, noise – therefore, heavenly powers – were categorized as yang. The opposite – that is, earthly powers, which make plants grow – are categorized as yin. The *I Ching*, the famous divination book, has been the bible of the Chinese for 5000 years. This is based on 64 hexagrams which consist of 8 trigrams. These 8 trigrams are combinations of nothing other than 3 yins or yangs. In the *I Ching*, yin is symbolized by a broken line (- -) while yang is symbolized by a straight line (—).

We can see such yin yang symbols everywhere and at any time. For examples see Table 13, p. 74.

There are several important concepts in the *I Ching*. 1. Yin and yang are antagonistic but also complementary. Therefore, the yin yang concept is not Western dualism which sees nature as two antagonisms: capitalist vs. labor, rich vs. poor, good vs. bad, right vs. wrong. Oriental dualism sees two forces which antagonize but at the same time are complementary. In the West, men and women are antagonistic; in the East they are complementary. Lao Tsu well expressed this complementarity in the *Tao Te Ching*, second chapter: "Under heaven, we all know beauty as beauty because there is ugliness. We know virtue because there are bad deeds." 2. There is yin inside yang, and there is yang inside yin. In other words, there is a seed of happiness when we are unhappy, and vice versa. There is a seed of sickness when we are healthy, and vice versa. 3. *I* (易) means change. Yin yang also means change. Yin changes to yang, and yang changes to yin. This concept is the result of the observation of seasonal changes. Therefore, this change is not lineal change, but cyclic change. There is no beginning and end. When this cyclic concept develops, the 5 element theory and 12 meridian theory develop.

Like the I Ching, another bible of the Chinese and one of the best selling philosophical books in this country is the Tao Te Ching, by Lao Tsu. Lao Tsu expresses that this world is made by the interaction of two forces - yin and yang. Since yin and yang are relative to each other, the yin value changes according to the change of the yang value; there is no absolute value, truth, or virtue in this world. The free man, or wisest man, therefore, lives with Tao, the order of the universe. In other words, he accepts any natural changes.

Chapter 22 is a poetic expression of Lao Tsu's yin yang philosophy:

> The imperfect becomes perfect;
> The crooked becomes straight.
> The empty will be filled;
> And old things renewed.
> He who has little will gain;
> He who has plenty loses.
> The man of supreme wisdom
> Clings to the Tao - the One
> And is ever free.
> But not clinging to his ego,
> He clearly perceives.
> Not stuck in opinion,
> His understanding is clear.
> Not proud of his deeds,
> He is honored.
> Not haughty in success,
> His fortune continues.
> Not competing in the relative world -
> Knowing it is quicksand - none can upset him.

Translation by Herman Aihara

According to the Chinese legend, in ancient China, Fu Hi made the *I Ching;* Shen Nung taught herbal therapy; and the Yellow Emperor Huang Ti compiled the *Nei Ching* – 'The Yellow Emperor's Classic of Internal Medicine.' The *I Ching* is a book on the principle of living, while the *Nei Ching* is a book on medicine, consisting of two parts. The first part is on the theory of medicine and the second part is on practical acupuncture treatment (further popularized in the U.S.A. after Nixon's visit to China). Shen Nung's work is the origin of Chinese herbal medicine. The basic concept of all this work is yin yang. Since I previously introduced the *I Ching,* I will translate some paragraphs from the *Nei Ching:*

"The yin and yang conditions of the four seasons are the foundation of all phenomena. Therefore, wise men warn us to perspire yang energy in spring and summer, while keeping energy in during the yin winter and autumn. Such is living in accordance with the Order of the Universe."

"Yin and yang antagonize and complement each other and from them all phenomena are produced; for example, day and night, and the cycle of four seasons. In other words, yin and yang are the father and mother of all changes. Yin yang is the cause of life and death. Yin yang is the manifestation of the creator. Therefore, curing sickness must be based on the principle of yin yang." [This is the basic principle of Chinese (or Oriental) medicine.]

In the case of character, yang means busy and active, while yin means calm and quiet. Yang is the foundation of germination and yin is the foundation of nourishment or growth.

Mao Tse Tung stated in his *On Contradiction:*

> In mathematics: plus and minus, differential and integral.

In mechanics: action and reaction.
In physics: positive and negative electricity.
In chemistry: the combination and dissociation
   of atoms.
In social science: the class structure.

What is more important is their transformation
into each other. That is to say, in a given condition,
each of the contradictory aspects within a thing
transform into the opposite.

All processes have a beginning and an end; all
processes transform themselves into their oppo-
sites.

We Chinese often say, "Things that oppose each
other also complement each other." That is, things
opposed to each other have identity. There is an
absolute in the relative.

In the Occident, there were also many yin yang
thinkers. The dialectical view of thought in the Western
world was developed by Hegel in the 19th century. However, it was Engels who developed the view of dialectics in
natural science. In *Dialectics of Nature* he says, "All natural
processes are two-sided; they rest on the relation of at
least two effective parts, action and reaction." It is interesting that Hegel says that in essence everything is relative. Ohsawa says, "There is no absolute yin or yang.
They are relative to each other."

It is important to point out that yin and yang is not a
concept of dualism such as most Western thinkers might
assume. The *Encyclopedia Britannica* defines dualism as
follows:

"Dualism is the doctrine that the world (or reality)
consists of two basic, opposed, and irreducible principles
or substances (i.e. good and evil; mind and matter) that
account for all that exists. It has played an important role
in the history of thought and religion." According to this

definition, the yin and yang concept seems to be dualism. However, yin and yang is not dualism. George Ohsawa stated that yin and yang are two sides of Oneness, which is the Creator of the Universe, God, Universal Consciousness, or whatever it may be called. Oneness is invisible. When this invisible reality manifests in this world, it appears as yin and yang, two antagonistic forces or phenomena. Therefore, yin and yang are relative manifestations of God or Universal Consciousness – man's monistic, invisible, and ultimate concept. This is very important because if one considers yin and yang another form of dualism, he is confusing gold with copper.

Ohsawa applied the yin yang concept to scientific fields such as physics, physiology, biology, medicine, chemistry, etc. In *The Book of Judgment*, he wrote:

> The Unique Principle divides all things into two antagonistic categories; yin and yang according to the Chinese wise men, or Tamasic and Rajasic or Shiva and Vishnu if one follows the Indian saints. They are, indeed, two complementary forces, indispensable each to the other, like man to woman, day to night. They are the two fundamental and opposite factors that continually produce, destroy and produce, repeatedly, all that exists in the universe.
>
> From the physical point of view, that which contains more water (every other condition being equal) is yin; the reverse is true of yang. According to the Unique Principle, everything may be classified in one or the other of the two categories, then coordinated in accordance with respective proportions of their yin and yang constituents.
>
> All the characteristics of things in this universe are functions of the proportions and of the way in which they combine yin and yang. In other words, all phenomena and the character of things are influenced by the two fundamental forces: the centripetal yang and the centrifugal yin.

Centripetal yang produces the following phenomena: heat (this, the activity of the molecular com-
ponents); constriction; density; heaviness, thus the
tendency to go downward; flattened, low horizontal forms. On the contrary, centrifugal yin produces: cold; dilation; expansion; lightness, thus the
tendency to go upward; enlargement, tall (in the
vertical sense) thin forms.

All that exists in this universe has a shape, color,
and characteristic weight. The lengthened form in
the vertical direction is yin, while the same form
horizontally is yang - the latter being under the
influence of the centripetal yang force, and the
former under the centrifugal yin.

All physical conditions are yin or yang. Table 11 shows
some physical conditions classified by yin and yang.

In climate or any material, hotter is more yang than
colder. Therefore, places near the equator have a yang
climate and the arctic has a yin climate. Hot water is more
yang than cold water and hot soup is more yang than cold,
other things being equal. Therefore, yang persons like a
colder soup while yin persons like a hot soup. However,
the hot climate produces yin vegetables and fruits, and
the cold climate produces yang ones.

According to Chinese medicine, the bitter taste is most
yang, the next is salty, and then sweet. Hot is the most yin
taste, and sour is next to yin. Since the sweet tastes are
most balanced, it is always desirable that cooked foods
taste sweet.

If the body muscle is hard, it is more yang. However,
sometimes there is an opposite case. For example, some-
one who has a very hard shoulder is usually very yin, if
the hardness of shoulders comes from deposits of excess
protein and fat, which are yin.

Heavier things are more yang, and lighter things are

Table 11. Yin Yang Classification by Physical Conditions

Yang						Yin

red	orange	yellow	green	blue	indigo	violet
hot		warm		cool		cold
bitter	salty		sweet	sour		hot (spicy)
solid		liquid		gas		plasma
heavy						light
active						quiet
contraction		coagulation		separation		expansion
moving downward					moving upward	
round, short, thick				oblong, flat, thin, long		
time						space
anger	joy	pleasure (peace)		sadness	resentfulness	
centripetal force					centrifugal force	
inside center					outer periphery	

Trigrams:

☰   ☷   ☳   ☶   ☵   ☴   ☲   ☷

(From *Natural Medicine*, George Ohsawa, 1938.)

yin. Heavier things go down faster, and lighter ones go down less easily or even go up.

Moving is a yang manifestation, while staying still is yin. However, there are opposite cases. For example, electrons are moving fast, but they are considered yin compared to protons, which do not move. In this case, electrons are yin because they are circling outside and have a negative charge. Protons are yang because they are situated at the center and are positively charged.

Contraction is yang because the centripetal force dominates. Expansion is yin because centrifugal force is dominant. Our heart continuously contracts and expands from birth to death without rest. If it rests, we call it a heart attack. In reality, it is not an attack: the heart is resting because we gave it too much work to do. The heart contracts and expands by the stimulation of the autonomic nervous system. In other words, the sympathetic nerve (yin) causes expansion (yin) and the parasympathetic nerve stops expansion and the heart muscle itself contracts. Yin foods cause more expansion and yang foods make contraction stronger. Many heart medicines are yin, so that they cause expansion and for awhile the heart beats stronger. However, if such yin medicine is continued, the heart becomes weaker. Digitalis is the only yang heart medicine.

A round or square face is more yang than an oblong or triangular face.

Defining time and space by yin and yang is one of the most interesting examples of the yin yang theory. Time is yang, whereas space is yin. In the great space of planets and interplanets, time is huge. The Milky Way is so big that it has a diameter of 200 million light years. You see, here space is measured by time in light years. In other words, time and space are two sides of one coin. We live in the present time which is so short – yang. However, space is expanding infinitely – therefore it is yin.

Our psychological conditions are connected with our physical conditions and are also explained by yin and yang. When you are angry, the body is tight, the fist is clenched – that is yang. When you are joyful and peaceful, the body is relaxed – that is yin. When resentful, which is extremely yin, the body is then tight again. In other words, with both extreme emotions (resentfulness, yin; or anger, yang) the body contracts, and tension is produced. A joyful and peaceful mind represents psychologically balanced yin and yang; this makes relaxation. The opposite is also true: a relaxed body encourages a peaceful mind.

All elements radiate specific wave lengths. According to Ohsawa, we can judge the yin and yang gradation by spectroscopic radiations. In other words, if elements produce a long wave radiation, they are yang. Such ele-ments are H (hydrogen), Na (sodium), C (carbon), and Li (lithium). If elements produce a short wave radiation, they are yin. Such elements are O (oxygen), N (nitrogen), P (phosphorus), and K (potassium).

According to Table 12, Na has a long wave radiation, so it is yang, and K has a short wave radiation, so it is yin; this confirms Ishizuka's theory.

Most living creature are richer in yin than in yang elements. Therefore, there is more K than Na in animals, as well as plants. Ishizuka set the ideal ratio of K:Na in man's foods as 5:1. Ohsawa wrote in *Natural Medicine* that this ratio can fluctuate between 3:2 to 7:1 for man, depending on his living environment. Ohsawa classified the yin and yang of foods by K:Na and K–Na. Therefore, I classify foods as yin and yang, using the ratio K:Na and difference K–Na.

4. Yin and Yang Foods

Thus far in this chapter, I have discussed the concept of yin and yang and its general use. Now I will discuss how to determine the yin and yang of foods. From a macrobiotic

Table 12. Yin Yang Classification of Elements by Spectroscopy

Red (above 6500 A°)	Orange (6499 to 6000 A°)	Yellow (5999 to 5750 A°)	Green (5749 to 4820 A°)	Blue (4819 to 4290 A°)	Violet (below 4289 A°)
Li H		He		Be	
C	Na	Ne		F	B
		Mg			O N
		Cl		P	Al Si
				S	
		Sc		A	
		Cr	Ti	V Ca	K
		Ni			Mn
				Fe	
			Cu		Co
			Zn		Ga
			Ge		
		As	Se		
			Br	Kr	Rb Sr
				Y	Zr
		Pd	In		Nb
		Ag	Cd	Rh	Ru Mo
		Te I	Cs	Xe	Sb
			Ba	Ce	La
			Sm	Nd	Pr
				Em	
				Tb	Eu
		In Ta		Dy	
		Pt Au		Ho	Er Tu
		Hg Tl		W	Os
		Th	Ra Bi		Pb

yang activity ———————————————————— yin activity

(From *The Unique Principle,* by George Ohsawa.)

Table 13. General Yin and Yang Classification

Symbol	Force	Energy	Atom	Element	Color	Season	Time of day
yin ▽ –					ultra-violet		
minus	centrifugal		electron	O, N		winter	
		magnetic			violet		midnight
							to
							dawn
				P, S			
		electric			indigo		
				K		autumn	dusk
Chinese yin yang					blue		to
							midnight
Jewish star		chemical			green		
			neutron				
Christian cross					yellow		
							dawn
					brown		to
						spring	noon
					orange		
		mechanical					
				Na			noon
					red		to
plus △ +			proton				dusk
yang	centripetal	gravitational, heat		H	infrared	summer	

Table 13. continued

Foods	Physical condition	Emotion	Psychological condition	Activity	Music
	weak pulse			sleep	
		cry	stubborn		
chemical					religious
additives	pale face		pessimist		
		worry		meditation	
processed			negative thinker		
foods	big, extruded eye				
			introvert		blues
fruits				writing	
	yellow face		listener		
vegetables					
		comfortable		cooking	
grains			good listener		country
	pink face		good talker	singing	
dairy				talking	
	small eye		talker	walking	
fish		joy			
poultry			extrovert	dancing	
pork	red face				rock & roll
beef		laughing	positive thinker	screaming	
eggs					
miso	strong pulse		optimist	disco	
soy sauce				dancing	disco
		anger	overconfident		
salt	good complexion			jogging	

point of view, there are two kinds of elements: yin elements and yang elements. Na is a yang element, and K, Fe, S, and P are yin elements. Yang foods are rich in Na and yin foods are rich in K, Fe, S, and/or P, relatively speaking. Magnesium (Mg) seems to stand almost in the middle of yin to yang, and might be slightly toward the yang side. Calcium (Ca) is very rich in fish, but not in beef, pork, or chicken. Ca is also very rich in beans and some vegetables, such as radish leaves, but not in grains. Therefore, Ca is not an element by which we can determine the yin or yang of foods. Since K is the most popular yin element and Na is the most popular yang element, Ohsawa used the ratio K:Na and the difference K – Na to determine the yin and yang of foods.

Rule 1: If the ratio K:Na is larger, it is more yin compared with one which has smaller K:Na.

Rule 2: If the ratio K:Na is smaller, then it is more yang compared with one which has a larger K:Na.

Rule 3: Larger K – Na means more yin than one which has a smaller K – Na value.

Rule 4: Smaller K – Na means more yang than one which has a larger K – Na value.

In Table 14, K:Na and K – Na of eggs are both small compared with other foods, so we may say eggs are very yang. In this table, codfish is the most yang. K:Na of carrot shows 1.8 – almost as yang as eggs. This happened, I suspect, due to an experimental error as to what part of the carrot was used for the measurements. Please check, using Table 15, for carrots. In order to confirm the validity of K:Na, and K – Na to determine yin and yang, I made a similar list of foods from two more recent books. This is Table 15. You see, the values of K:Na and K – Na in Table 15 are much larger than those in Table 14. This shows, I

Table 14. K and Na Contents around 1930
(100 gr. samples)

Foods	K (mg.)	Na (mg.)	K:Na	K - Na
codfish	22.0	59.0	0.4	-37.0
eggs, chicken	17.4	22.9	0.8	-5.5
egg white	31.4	31.6	1.0	-0.2
sea bass	21.0	19.0	1.1	-2.0
egg yolk	9.3	5.9	1.6	3.4
barley	16.8	4.2	4.0	12.6
carrots	36.5	20.7	1.8	15.8
rye	18.3	1.5	12.2	16.8
buckwheat	23.5	6.1	3.9	17.4
brown rice	23.0	4.6	5.0	18.4
millet	23.7	4.1	5.8	19.6
wheat	31.0	1.7	16.0	29.3
white rice	28.0	2.0	14.0	26.0
radishes	34.7	14.3	2.8	20.4
human milk	33.8	9.2	3.5	24.6
meat	36.9	9.6	4.0	27.3
tea	37.6	8.0	4.5	29.6
onions	34.7	2.8	12.0	31.9
lotus root	47.6	14.3	3.3	33.3
cabbage	44.3	8.3	5.1	36.0
soybeans	44.4	1.0	44.0	43.4
pears	52.9	8.8	6.0	44.1
grapes	50.0	5.0	10.0	45.0
peanuts	47.9	1.2	40.0	46.7
mushrooms	54.3	5.0	11.0	49.3
sweet potatoes	54.3	3.3	16.5	51.0
apples	55.9	3.0	18.0	52.9
eggplant	54.3	1.4	39.0	52.9
potatoes	60.4	3.1	20.0	57.3
bamboo shoots	62.5	4.2	14.9	58.3
coffee	261.0	6.0	44.0	255.0

(From *Natural Medicine*, George Ohsawa, 1938.)

Table 15. K and Na Contents around 1970
(100 gr. samples)

Foods	K (mg.)	Na (mg.)	K:Na	K - Na
almonds, unsalted	690	3	230	687
apples, fresh w/skin	110	1	110	109
asparagus, raw	278	2	139	276
avocados, raw	604	4	151	600
bacon, cured, raw	57	253	0.23	-196
bananas, raw	370	1	370	369
barley, pearl	336	7.5	44.8	328.5
bass, sea, fresh	256	68	3.8	188
bean curds, fried (age)	100	14	7.1	86
beans, azuki	1500	20	70	1480
beans, black	1300	4	325	1296
beans, lima, raw	650	2	325	648
beans, pinto, raw	984	10	98	974
beans, red, raw	984	10	98	974
beans, soy	1680	3	560	1677
beans, white, raw	1198	19	63	1178
beef cuts, lean	603	48.8	12.4	554
broccoli, raw	382	15	25.5	367
cabbage, head, raw	233	20	11.7	213
(Chinese cabbage has about the same value as the above.)				
carp, raw, white	286	50	5.7	236
carrots, raw, w/o tops	341	47	7.3	294
cashews	465	15	31	450
catfish fillet, raw	330	60	5.5	270
caviar, sturgeon	180	2200	0.08	-2020
celery, raw	341	126	2.7	215
cheese, cottage	85	229	0.37	-144
cheese, cheddar	82	700	0.12	-618
(Swiss cheese is a little more yin than cheddar cheese; processed American cheese is much more yang.)				
chestnuts	1140	16	71	1124
chickpeas	797	26	30.7	771
chocolate, w/o sugar	831	4	208	827

Table 15. continued

Foods	K (mg.)	Na (mg.)	K:Na	K - Na
codfish, raw, whole	382	70	5.5	312
coffee, roasted, whole	1600	2	800	1598
corn, kernel, raw	202	1	202	201
cucumber, whole	160	6	27	154
dandelion greens	398	76	5.2	322
dates, domestic	638	1	638	637
egg white, fresh	139	152	.91	-13
egg yolk, fresh	112	71	1.6	41
eggs, chicken, raw, whole	130	122	1.1	8

(The white of an egg is most yang; next is the whole egg; and the least is the yolk. They are all too yang with almost no yin; therefore, one who eats eggs every day will have troubles such as heart disease.)

Foods	K (mg.)	Na (mg.)	K:Na	K - Na
eggplant, raw	214	2	207	212
figs, raw	194	2	97	192
flour, buckwheat	260	14	19	246
flour, wheat	140	5	28	135
garlic	528	19	27.8	509
grapefruit, raw	135	1	135	134
halibut, raw	449	54	8.3	395
lentils, dry	790	30	26.3	760
milk, cow, whole	144	50	2.9	94
milk, goat	180	34	5.3	146
milk, human	51	16	3.2	35
miso	545	5100	0.11	-4555
mushrooms, raw	414	15	27.6	399
mustard greens, raw	377	32	11.8	345
noodles, egg	136	5.5	25	130
noodles, soba, boiled	30	90	0.33	-60
noodles, udon, boiled	5	17	0.29	-12
onion, raw	157	10	15.7	147
orange	200	1	200	219
oyster, eastern	121	73	1.7	48
parsley	727	45	16	682
peanuts, raw	676	5.3	128	671
pork, raw	360	51	7.1	671

Table 15. continued

Foods	K (mg.)	Na (mg.)	K:Na	K-Na
potatoes, albi	540	10	54	530
potatoes, raw	407	3.0	136	404
potatoes, sweet	330	40	8.3	290
pumpkin, raw	340	1	340	339
radishes, no tops	321	18	18.3	303
raisins, dried	763	27	28.3	736
rice, brown, raw	112	4	28	108
salmon, king, fresh	399	45	8.9	354
seaweed, dulse	8071	2088	3.87	5983
seaweed, kelp	5280	3011	1.75	2269
seaweed, kombu	6600	2700	2.4	3900
seaweed, nori	3800	680	5.6	3120
seaweed, wakame	2700	2540	1.1	160
sesame seeds, dry	726	60	12.1	666
shrimp	220	140	1.6	80
soy sauce	457	8367	0.05	-7910
spaghetti, enriched	195	2	97	193
spinach, raw	470	71	6.6	399
squash, summer, raw	202	1	202	201
strawberries, raw	164	1	164	163
sugar, black	630	13	48.5	617
taro, raw	514	7	73.4	507
tomatoes, ripe, raw	244	3	81.3	241
vinegar, cider	100	1.1	100	99
walnuts	573	3	191	570
watercress, raw	282	52	5.4	230
wheat, whole, red, spring	370	3.1	119	367
yeast, baker's dry	2000	52	38	1948
yeast, brewer's	1896	121	16	1775
yoghurt, skimmed milk	132	47	2.8	85

(From *Food Values of Portions Commonly Used,* by Bowes and Church; and *Food Composition,* by the Japanese Government Department of Science and Technology.)

believe, that foods are generally becoming more yin due to the fact that much more fertilizers and chemicals are used now than before.

Highly processed foods or drinks in Table 15, such as most commercial foods and beer or wine, should not be relied on. If beer or wine is made in a very natural way, the value will be much different than we have here.

Generally speaking, the following classification can be applied:

	Very yin	Well balanced	Very yang
K:Na	over 100	100-10	less than 10
K - Na	over 200	200-100	less than 100

Any grains that are milled or floured lose most of their sodium, and are very yinnized.

Broccoli, cabbage, carrots, cashews, celery, garlic, mushrooms, mustard greens, parsley, raisins, seaweed, spinach, watercress, yeast, and yoghurt have small values of K:Na, and it means that these are very yang. However, the K - Na values of these foods are quite large and it means these are yin. Therefore, we have to decide the yin and yang of foods not only by K:Na and K - Na, but also by other factors, such as the following:

a. Vegetables which grow bigger or more abundantly in the south are yin; those that grow bigger or more abundantly in the north are yang (this is in the Northern Hemisphere).

b. In the Northern Hemisphere, vegetables which grow from April to September are yin and between October and March are yang.

c. Vegetables which grow vertically above the earth are yin; those that grow horizontally are yang.

d. Vegetables which grow horizontally under the earth are yin; those which grow vertically are yang.

e. Vegetables which grow faster are yin and those that grow slower are yang.

f. Vegetables which grow taller are yin and those that grow shorter are yang.

g. Vegetables which can be cooked in a shorter time are yin; the ones that take longer are yang. There are, however, exceptions for this in cooking. Some yang vegetables such as jinenjo (natural long potato), green scallions, and celery do not need long cooking. All beans take a long time to cook, yet they are yin.

h. Violet, indigo, blue, green, or white colors are signs of yin vegetables; yellow, orange, brown, red, and black are signs of yang vegetables. However, there are exceptions for this too; tomatoes have a red color, but they are yin (acidic and watery).

i. Watery vegetables are yin and drier ones are yang.

j. Heavier vegetables are yang, lighter ones are yin.

k. Soft vegetables are yin and harder ones are yang. (If you want sweeter squash, buy heavier and harder ones.)

To distinguish the yin and yang of animal foods is not so important because we don't recommend animal foods much anyway. We eat them occasionally. However, for the beginners who still want to eat them, and/or for those who want to study the yin and yang of foods, here I will show you a few general rules.

a. Warmblooded animal foods are more yang than coldblooded ones. Therefore, beef, pork, chicken and fowl are more yang than fish (shell-fish, etc.). This is one of the reasons we recommend fish or shellfish more than warm-blooded animals and meats. Processed fish, however, often has a high Na content due to the addition of salt, which makes these foods too yang.

b. In the Northern Hemisphere, animals that grow bigger in the South (warmer climate) are yin and those that grow bigger in the North (colder climate) are yang.

c. Hibernating animals are yin; those that do not hibernate are yang.

d. Animals of slow movement are yin; fast and active ones are yang.

e. Saltwater fish are more yang than freshwater fish.

Fish that live at the bottom of the water (either ocean, lake, or river) are more yin than ones that live near the surface of the water. For example, carp live at the bottom of the river or lake, where there is less oxygen than at the surface. Carp require less oxygen because their blood holds much oxygen. This is the reason carp blood is given to pneumonia patients in the Orient.

Table 16 shows the ratio and difference between K and Na in various body fluids.

Many natural food dieters use honey instead of white sugar or saccharin. Honey is more natural and contains vitamins, so of course is a much better food than sugar or saccharin. From the macrobiotic point of view, however, the use of honey must be moderate because it is a very yin

Table 16. Comparison of K and Na in Various Body Fluids

Name of fluid	K mg./ml.	Na	K:Na	K-Na	
Blood plasma (alkaline)	91	350	0.26	-259	(yang)
Saliva (alkaline)	76	76	1.00	0	(yang)
Sweat (alkaline)	39	134	0.29	-95	(yang)
Pancreatic juice (alkaline)	18	324	0.06	-306	(yang)
Intestinal juice (alkaline)	90	249	0.38	-150	(yang)
Stomach juice (acid)	36	136	0.26	-100	(yang)
Urine (alkaline)	195	207	0.94	-12	(yang)
Stool	282	81	3.48	201	(yin)

Table 17. Quantity of Various Elements in Human Blood and Bee Honey

Element	Human Blood mg./ml.	Bee Honey mg./ml.
K	0.030	0.3860
Na	0.320	0.0010
Mg	0.018	0.0180
S	0.004	0.0010
P	0.005	0.0019
Fe	trace	0.0007
Ca	0.011	0.0040
Cl	0.360	0.0290
I	trace	trace
K:Na	1:10 (0.03:0.32)	386:1 0.386:0.001)

food. Look at Table 17. (I cannot show you the source of this information, because I no longer have the book.)

The elemental composition of honey is amazingly similar to that of human blood, except for the K and Na contents. The ratio of K (yin) to Na (yang) in human blood is 1 to 10, while the same ratio in honey is 386 to 1. Therefore, honey is 4000 times more yin than human blood.

Using the above-mentioned yin and yang concepts, we can classify all foods into yin and yang categories. Such classification has been made by many macrobiotic students. I did one in *The Dō of Cooking* which is shown here as Table 18 (p. 86).

Table 18. Yin Yang Classification of Various Foods

Fruits
tropical
lemons
peaches
pears
oranges
watermelon
apples
strawberries

Seaweeds
nori
hijiki
wakame
kombu

Nuts & Seeds
cashews
peanuts
almonds
chestnuts

squash
pumpkin
sunflower
sesame

Beans
soybeans
green peas
white
pinto
kidney
black
chickpeas
azuki

Beverages
sugared drinks
fruit juices
coffee
tea (dyed)
mineral water
soda water
deep well water
kokkoh
bancha tea
mu tea
yannoh
ginseng

Animal Foods
shellfish
white meat fish
fowl
meat
red meat fish
eggs

Alcoholic Beverages
vodka
wine
whiskey
sake
beer

Vegetables
potatoes
eggplant
tomatoes
shiitake
taro potatoes
cucumber
sweet potatoes
spinach
asparagus
celery
cabbage
pumpkin
onions
garlic
turnips
daikon
lotus root
burdock
carrots

jinenjo

Grains
corn
oats
barley
rye
wheat
rice
millet
buckwheat

Dairy Foods
ice cream
yoghurt
butter
milk

goat's milk

soft cheeses
hard cheeses

Condiments
gomashio

tamari
miso

salt

Foods are listed from yin (top) to yang (bottom). This chart is only a guide since origin, manner of growth or production, season, the part of the food used, manner of cooking, etc., affect their yin and yang qualities.

CHAPTER V

Four Wheel Balance of Foods

1. Acid and Alkaline/Yin and Yang Classification of Foods

Having presented foods in terms of both their yin yang tendencies and their acid and alkaline forming characteristics, I am ready to bring the two approaches together. Acid forming foods can be classified yin or yang according to their content of sodium (Na), potassium (K), calcium (Ca), magnesium (Mg), phosphorus, (P), and sulfur (S). Alkaline forming foods can also be classified yin or yang, in the same manner.

Yin acid forming foods are high in P and S but not in Na. Yang acid forming foods are high in P, S, and Na.

Yin alkaline forming foods are high in K and Ca but not in P and S. Yang alkaline forming foods are high in Na and Mg but not in P and S.

Therefore, all foods can be classified into four sections (like the four wheels of a car), as follows in Table 19.

2. How to Read the Four-Wheel Chart

I have classified chemicals, medicinal drugs, psychedelic drugs, white sugar, candy, soft drinks, commercial vinegar, saccharin, and all refined foods as acid forming

Table 19. Food Comparison in Relation to
Yin Yang and Acid Alkaline

Section II Yin acid forming foods	Section I Yin alkaline forming foods
chemical drugs, pills sugar, candy, soft drinks alcohol drinks beans, nuts	honey, coffee herb tea, bancha tea fruits, seeds vegetables
Section IV Yang acid forming foods	Section III Yang alkaline forming foods
grains animal foods	radish pickle, dry soy sauce miso, salted umeboshi salt

foods. The reason for this is as follows. These foods are lacking in minerals, especially alkaline forming minerals. Therefore when these foods are eaten our body cannot neutralize the acid which is created by them unless stored alkaline forming minerals are used. In other words, since these foods bring no alkaline forming minerals with them, their digestion will eliminate alkaline forming minerals stored in our body. This is the reason that these foods are classified as acid forming foods even though they may not contain acid forming minerals. For this same reason, I also consider tofu to be an acid forming food because tofu is made of refined soybeans and is lacking in alkaline forming elements.

Even though most nutritionists consider unrefined

soybeans to be a strong alkaline forming food, I have classified them as an acid forming food. I think that soybeans - as well as other beans - are acid forming foods because they contain much fat and protein, both of which are acid forming. The reason for this is as follows. If we consume an excess amount of fat, at least some of the excess will be incompletely digested, and this incomplete burning of a fat produces acetic acid. This causes a condition of the body fluid which is too acid. The strong body odor which some people have is usually caused by the acetic acid in their systems.

In the case of protein, if we consume more protein than we need, the excess breaks down to produce blood urea nitrogen. Since urea has a diuretic effect on our systems, high levels of it in our blood cause the kidneys to excrete too much water. Along with this excess excretion of water, minerals such as calcium, sodium, and potasium are lost in the urine. Since those minerals are alkaline forming elements, we can say that one of the results of excess protein consumption is a rise in the acidity of body fluid. For this reason I have placed beans and bean products among the acid forming foods.

3. Balancing Meals

Balanced meals means that they are balanced with yin and yang factors as well as acid and alkaline factors. In Table 20, such foods can be chosen using the sections diagonally. For example, make a menu with yang acid forming foods (Section IV) and yin alkaline forming foods (Section I). Such meals are combinations of grains and vegetables, fish and salad, chicken and fruits. However, meals containing four kinds of foods picked out from each section of Table 19 or 20 will be better balanced. For

Table 20. Detail of Foods from Table 19

Section II
Yin Acid Forming Foods

most chemicals
medicinal drugs
psychedelic drugs
sugar
candy
soft drinks
vinegar
saccharin
vodka
some wine
whiskey   corn oil
sake   olive oil
beer   sesame oil
                                           peanut butter
soybeans   cashews   sesame butter
green peas   peanuts
tofu   almonds
white beans   chestnuts
pinto beans
kidney beans
black beans
chickpeas
red beans (azuki)

macaroni
spaghetti   huma

Section IV   cow
Yang Acid Forming Foods

corn, oats
barley, rye,
wheat
rice   shellfish
buckwheat   eel, carp
                    white meat fish
                    cheese
                    fowl
                    meat
                    tuna, salmon
                    eggs

Table 20. continued

Section I
Yin Alkaline Forming Foods

natural wine
natural sake
cola   honey   tropical fruits
cocoa   mustard   dates, figs
fruit juices   ginger   lemons, grapes
coffee   pepper   raisins, bananas
tea (dyed)   curry   peaches
mineral water   cinnamon   currants   potatoes
soda water   pears, plums   eggplant
well water   oranges   tomatoes
                                watermelon   shiitake
                                apples, cherries   taro potatoes
                                strawberries   cucumber
                                                      sweet potatoes
                                                      mushrooms
                                                      spinach
                                                      asparagus
                                                      broccoli
                                                      celery
                                                      cabbage
                                                      pumpkin
                                                      onions
                                                      turnips
                  squash seeds   daikon
                  pumpkin seeds   nori
                  sunflower seeds   hijiki
milk   sesame seeds   carrots

milk

Section III
Yang Alkaline Forming Foods

kuzu tea
                                                wakame
                                                kombu
                                                lotus root
                  millet   burdock
dandelion tea   dandelion root
mu tea   jinenjo
Ohsawa coffee   sesame salt
yannoh   soy sauce
ginseng   miso
                  umeboshi
                  salt

example, such a balanced menu would include miso, grains, vegetables, and beans.

Generally speaking, for yang persons it is advisable to take 50% or more of Sections I and II. For yin persons, take 50% or more of Sections III and IV. This is a very general guideline for healthy and normally active persons. For sick persons, I recommend reading *Practical Guide to Far Eastern Macrobiotic Medicine* (G.O.M.F.). Individual diet, one's constitution, past diet, environmental condition of living, activity, job, and age should all be considered. However, in most cases, if we select foods from a good cross section, they will be balanced.

Such selection of foods is intuitive and traditional. For example, a big steak (Section IV) will be accompanied by plenty of salads, fruits, and wine (Section I). If you crave sugar, you better cut down your salt intake. This salt may come not only from table salt, but also from processed foods or meat.

The morning after a dinner party where one has eaten lots of beef, chicken, or cheese, one wants lots of coffee or oranges. Meat eaters wake up with a cup of coffee or orange juice. This is balancing not only yin and yang, but also acid and alkaline.

Office workers often take coffee breaks because working causes acid in the bloodstream. Coffee will help them to alkalize. However, coffee is very yin, so it is not recommended for vegetarians. For vegetarians, twig tea or mu tea will be a better alkaline forming drink.

You may like to serve a dinner with rice, fish, tofu and beer. This will be well balanced from the standpoint of yin and yang; however, these are all acid forming foods. Therefore it is not balanced in the end. You should add plenty of radish, leafy greens, tea, or fruits (optional for yang persons).

These tables (19 and 20) will be a great help for housewives when selecting menus.

The macrobiotic diet recommends grains (yang acid forming) as a main food. When combined with vegetables (yin alkaline forming) and salt (yang alkaline forming), the acid produced by the grain is balanced. Normally, 50-70% grains, 30-50% vegetables (including seaweed and beans), and salt (including soy sauce, miso, salty pickles) will balance the acid and alkaline factors in the blood.

People who have eaten animal food for a long time tend to have high blood acidity, even though they may have stored large amounts of alkaline forming elements in the form of sodium in their tissue. This sodium, stored in the tissues, is not ionized in the blood, however, and the blood remains acid. In this situation, alkaline forming foods in the form of vegetables and fruits, and only a small amount of grains, are required in the diet. Such a person cannot take much sodium as an alkaline forming element. Kanten (seaweed jello), wakame, nori, kombu, and hijiki are good for such persons.

In macrobiotics, some yin and yang acid forming foods are not recommended but most of the alkaline forming foods are recommended. In the macrobiotic diet, grains are the most acid forming foods; the rest of the diet consists of predominately alkaline forming foods. Therefore, there should be no trouble with acid alkaline balance when the foods are selected according to yin and yang – except when following a rigid grain-only diet. From the standpoint of acid and alkaline, then, most Americans should not start with a grain-only diet.

However, when one chews thoroughly – 100 to 200 times per mouthful – the acid grains become alkaline by mixing with the alkaline salivary enzyme ptyalin, and thus do not create acidity even if one eats only grains. Please read the following books to improve balanced meals:

The Calendar Cookbook – Cornellia Aihara
The Dō of Cooking – Cornellia Aihara
Macrobiotic Kitchen – Cornellia Aihara
Macrobiotic Cuisine – Lima Ohsawa
Complete Guide to Macrobiotic Cooking – Aveline Kushi
Cooking with Miso – Aveline Kushi
Introduction to Macrobiotic Cooking – Wendy Esko
Cooking with Care and Purpose – Michel Abehsera
The Book of Whole Meals – Annemarie Colbin

CHAPTER VI

Acid and Alkaline in Life

1. Acidosis

Acidosis is the tendency towards overacidity that arises in certain diseases. Acid is always developing in the body but it is usually carried away in the body's excretions.

There are some conditions affecting the digestion in which acidosis develops either because of increased acid production or because of the loss of alkaline substances by way of the bowels. This happens when there is much loss of fluid from vomiting or diarrhea. The treatment is to replace the lost fluid and to hinder the production of acid substances by giving water and salts. Macrobiotics recommends the following drinks to treat diarrhea or vomiting:

1) Sho-ban (soy sauce and bancha twig tea)
2) Salt plum, ginger, soy sauce, bancha tea
3) Seaweed soup
4) Miso soup with wakame
5) Kuzu, soy sauce, salt plum, bancha tea

Diabetes is the most common disease which causes acidosis. In diabetes, the body is unable to use glucose, so that fats are incompletely burned and acid substances are produced. The acid becomes accumulated if there are not enough alkaline forming substances in the blood.

Acidosis also develops in some diseases of the kidneys, but it is never as severe as in conditions associated with diabetes. Excess acid production in the stomach can also cause acidosis. This is the result of eating too much meat or refined grain; excessive work without good breathing; worry; indulgence in alcohol or tobacco; etc. Stomach ulcers are often associated with this condition.

Macrobiotic recommendations for excess acid caused by eating too much animal food, grain, or oily food include:

1) Wakame miso soup
2) Azuki bean rice
3) Daikon, cucumber, cabbage pickles
4) Boiled spinach
5) Grated radish
6) No animal food, no sugar

Western nutritionists have recommended citrus fruits as a natural cure for acidosis; this will be good if the acidosis is a result of excess animal food consumption.

The major effect of acidosis is depression of the central nervous system. When the pH of the blood falls below 7.0, the nervous system becomes so depressed that the person first becomes disoriented and finally comatose. Therefore, patients dying of diabetic acidosis, uremic acidosis, and other types of acidosis usually die in a state of coma. In acidosis, the high hydrogen ion (H^+) concentration causes an increased rate and depth of respiration. Therefore, one of the diagnostic signs of acidosis is increased pulmonary ventilation (rapid breathing). However, there is another type of acidosis that is manifested by slow breathing: this causes less carbon dioxide to be discharged and leads to an accumulation of carbonic acid in the blood.

In the case of acidosis caused by diabetes, kidney trouble,

and ulcers, animal food and sugar should be eliminated from the diet because they are a primary cause of acidity. Cooked grains and vegetables with a little salt, soy sauce, and miso should be the main diet. Externally, ginger compresses and albi plasters, or green plasters, can be applied to the kidneys for their improvement. (For these treatments, please read *Practical Guide to Far Eastern Macrobiotic Medicine,* by George Ohsawa.)

2. Alkalosis

Alkalosis is the opposite of acidosis. According to Guyton in *Medical Physiology:*

> Metabolic alkalosis does not occur nearly so often as metabolic acidosis. It most frequently follows excessive ingestion of alkaline drugs, such as sodium bicarbonate, for the treatment of gastritis or peptic ulcer. However, metabolic alkalosis occasionally results from *excessive vomiting of gastric contents* without vomiting of lower gastrointestinal contents, which causes excessive loss of the hydrochloric acid secreted by the stomach mucosa. The net result is loss of acid from the extracellular fluids and development of metabolic alkalosis. . . .
>
> The major effect of alkalosis on the body is *overexcitability of the nervous system.* This effect occurs both in the central nervous system and in the peripheral nerves, but usually the peripheral nerves are affected before the central nervous system. The nerves become so excitable that they automatically and repetitively fire even when they are not stimulated by normal stimuli. As a result, the muscles go into a stage of *tetany,* which means a state of tonic spasm. This tetany usually appears first in the muscles of the forearm, then spreads rapidly to the muscles of the face, and finally all over the body.

Alkalotic patients may die from tetany of the respiratory muscles. . . .

Only occasionally does an alkalotic person develop severe symptoms of central nervous system overexcitability. The symptoms may manifest themselves as extreme nervousness or, in susceptible persons, as convulsions. For instance, in persons who are predisposed to epileptic fits, simply overbreathing often results in an attack.

3. What Are the Acid Drugs?

Commonly, psychedelic drugs are called 'acid.' Are they truly acid? As the name suggests, LSD (lysergic acid diethylamide), mescaline (3, 4, 5 – trimethosyphenethylamine), and STP (2, 5 – dimethoxy – 4 methyl amphetamine) are all acid; they give off hydrogen ions (H^+). However, this does not mean they produce acid in our bodies. Those drugs, if not synthetic, belong to the alkaloid family.

According to *Collier's Encyclopedia*:

The term 'alkaloid,' meaning alkali-like, was first used by W. Meissner in 1821. Pierre Joseph Pelletier, who discovered quinine in 1820, initially used the suffix '-ine' as a distinctive ending for alkaloidal names. . . . The German ending '-in' is retained in such alkaloid names as 'heroin' and 'stypticin.' Most specific alkaloids receive their names from the scientific name of the plant (thus, aconitine from the generic name *Aconitum*), from the vernacular name of the plant or product (thus, quinine from the Spanish *quina*, meaning 'cinchona,' and ergonovine from the French *ergot*, 'spur'), from some physiological property (thus, morphine from the Latin *Morpheus*, the god of sleep, so named because of the drug's hypnotic properties), or from the name of a notable person (thus, pelletierine from the chemist Pelletier).

According to the *Encyclopedia Britannica*, alkaloids ". . . are notable chiefly for their physiological activity; many have long histories as poisons, narcotics, hallucinogens, and medicinal agents. Generally, alkaloids are basic, or alkaline, substances – i. e., they neutralize acids; their molecules contain chiefly atoms of carbon, hydrogen, and nitrogen, which is the source of their basicity."

The reason alkaloid drugs are alkaline is that they contain the alkaline forming element nitrogen, N. Why then are they not alkaline when they are synthetic? This is my claim, although I have not found scientific reports on this. The reason is that not only nitrogen, but other alkaline forming elements such as K, Na, Ca, and Mg exist in natural alkaloids. However, those elements are missing in the case of synthetic alkaloids. In my opinion, K, Na, Ca, and Mg are the elements which make the alkaloids alkaline.

According to *The Britannica*:

> The physiological activity of alkaloids is of importance not only in medicine but also in agriculture and in forensic chemistry. Narcotics addiction and the use of alkaloids as hallucinogens are major social problems. In medicine, alkaloids are employed as narcotics, analgesics; antimalarials; local anesthetics; as cardiac, uterine, and respiratory stimulants; and as materials that raise the blood pressure; cause the pupils to dilate; or bring about relaxation of the skeletal muscles. . . .
>
> Many alkaloids are of medical importance because they are the cause of occasional poisoning of livestock or man. [Some of them are henbane, nightshade, and thorn apple. These poisonous

plants belong to the Solanaceae family, which also includes the potato.] Another example is the group of ergot alkaloids, produced by a fungus (ergot) that grows on cereal grains; it finds legitimate use in medicine, but the ingestion of cereals containing ergot was the source of much serious illness (ergotism) until the cause was well understood.

For analgesic drugs, we have morphine, codeine and heroin (deacetylmorphine). If they did not exist, many movies and TV shows we have now would not have been created.

The Britannica continues:

> The cinchona alkaloid quinidine is the cardiac stimulant used to correct arrhythmias of the auricle (one of the chambers of the heart), and cinchona and rauwolfia alkaloids are used for arrhythmias of the ventricle (the other chamber of the heart). There are no generally acceptable alkaloids for congestive heart failure, in which the pumping action of the heart is inadequate though its rhythm is normal. Generally, another type of material, the digitalis glycosides, is the drug of choice for this kind of heart disease. . . .
>
> Many alkaloids influence respiration; virtually all of them, however, produce other, and often unwanted, effects. Atropine, for example, stimulates respiration in moderate doses, even when respiration has been depressed by morphine, but it also has a number of effects on the brain and dilates the pupils of the eyes. . . .
>
> Ergonovine, one of the ergot alkaloids, finds extensive use in obstetrics to reduce uterine hemorrhage following childbirth, its action being primarily constriction of the blood vessels. Ephedrine also causes constriction of blood vessels and, because of this action, it is widely used to alleviate the discomfort of common colds, sinusitis, hay fever, and

bronchial asthma. . . . The pupil-dilating action of ephedrine, unlike that of atropine, does not abolish the light reflexes and the accommodation reflexes of the eye. There are a number of other useful dilators and, of these, scopolamine is one of the more powerful. Cocaine, a potent local anesthetic, is also a dilator.

"Many alkaloids possess local anesthetic characteristics, and some of them do not produce the undesirable effects of cocaine. . . . Modern synthetic local anesthetics, cheaper and often superior to cocaine, have largely, but not entirely, displaced the alkaloid.

The mechanism of the physiological functions of the above-mentioned alkaloids can be explained by the yin yang principle. Those alkaloids (including synthetic ones) are very yin substances. Since they are yin, they stimulate the sympathetic nerve after entering the bloodstream. This sympathetic nerve produces the yin hormone called norepinephrine which stimulates yang organs such as the heart, liver, kidney, and lung. (Yin stimulant expands yang organs.) However, this stimulation causes blood vessel constriction, as mentioned above. Why? In reality, the blood vessel muscle is not contracting – it is expanding inwardly. Therefore, the result is constriction. Table 21 will show the antagonistic functions of the parasympathetic (yang) and sympathetic (yin) nerves. The parasympathetic nerve (yang) can be stimulated by yang drugs (if they exist) or foods such as miso, soy sauce, salt, etc. The sympathetic nerve (yin) can be stimulated by yin drugs (most drugs are); foods such as all fruits, most vegetables, spices, soft drinks, sugar, honey, and candies; and alcoholic drinks, coffee, and tea.

Those alkaloids are so yin that they neutralize Na in the extracellular fluid of the central and peripheral nerves.

Table 21. Automatic Effect on Various Organs
of the Body

Organs	Effect of Sympathetic Stimulation	Effect of Parasympathetic Stimulation
Eye: Pupil	Dilated	Contracted
Ciliary muscle	None	Excited
Sweat glands	Copious sweating (cholinergic)	None
Apocrine glands	Thick, odoriferous secretion	None
Heart: Muscle	Increased rate	Slowed rate
	Increased force of beat	Decreased force of beat
Coronaries	Vasodilated	Constricted
Lungs: Bronchi	Dilated	Constricted
Blood vessels	Mildly constricted	None
Liver	Glucose released	None
Gall bladder and bile ducts	Inhibited	Excited
Kidney	Decreased output	None
Ureter	Inhibited	Excited
Bladder: Detrusor	Inhibited	Excited
Trigone	Excited	Inhibited
Penis	Ejaculation	Erection
Blood vessels: Abdominal	Constricted	None
Muscle	Constricted (adrenergic) Dilated (cholinergic)	None
Skin	Constricted (adrenergic) Dilated (cholinergic)	Dilated
Blood: Coagulation	Increased	None
Glucose	Increased	None
Basal metabolism	Increased up to 50%	None
Adrenal cortical secretion	Increased	None
Mental activity	Increased	None
Pilo-erector muscles	Excited	None

(From *Function of the Human Body*, Guyton.)

As a result, our nervous system loses its polarity. Electricity is not created and communication stops. Thus alkaloids cause relief of pain, local anesthetic action, muscle relaxation, and even hallucination or euphoria (release of tension in the mind). The synthetic drugs can cause those yin effects but also cause acidity of blood. Natural drugs have fewer side effects.

Drugs, either natural or synthetic, affect not only the nervous systems; they also change brain functioning. They do this by blocking the effect of serotonin, though the exact mechanism of this is not known to present-day science. This effect is stronger if the drugs are synthetic.

From the macrobiotic point of view, psychedelic drugs have both strong alkaline and strong acid forming elements. The alkaline forming elements circulate downwards in the bloodstream, and the acid forming elements go up to the brain; thus the two vital factors of internal equilibrium separate in our bodies. In other words, affected by the alkalinity, our sensorial nervous system is excited and sends many stimuli to the brain, but the brain is inhibited by the acidity and is not able to assemble or collate the messages. The result is hallucinations.

Due to the high concentrations of acid, prolonged use of such drugs inevitably causes brain damage. The abuse of such drugs can be prevented by simply reducing the intake of sugar and animal foods (strong acid forming foods) because these foods are the cause of the attraction to drugs. (For more information: Ohsawa, Aihara, and Pulver, *Smoking, Marijuana and Drugs.*)

4. Dietary Advice in the Recovery from Sickness Caused by Taking Drugs

One who is suffering physically or mentally from the

effects of drugs must patiently and wisely first rebuild his health, because there is no miraculous cure for these sufferings. Whenever I meet young people who are suffering physically and mentally through years of drug use, I think and search for a cure. The following is my sincere advice to those who wish to reestablish their health and well-being.

Drugs damage the intestinal flora. Therefore, one who has abused drugs for a long time should not restrict his diet too narrowly. (Please read *Macrobiotics: An Invitation to Health and Happiness,* by George Ohsawa.) Rice bran pickles and miso soup will help to build up intestinal flora. Eat rice bran nuka pickles at every meal and miso soup once a day. (See *The Calendar Cookbook* or *Dō of Cooking* for making rice bran pickles.)

One who has weak intestines should chew well, eat whole grains, vegetables, seaweeds, and beans – all well cooked. It is often helpful to avoid breads, since their roughage is much harsher and more irritating to sensitive intestinal linings. Many friends who have taken much sugar or drugs have experienced intestinal hemorrhaging with breads. For such persons, softer forms of grains are better, such as noodles and some soups made with seaweeds. The Japanese varieties of seaweeds – kombu and wakame – are especially good for yinnized intestines because they have a mucilagenous quality which makes them very soothing and healing for the damaged intestines. They also provide large amounts of minerals which help alkalize the blood. This effect is very important because many drug takers tend to have an acidic condition even though the first reaction from drugs seems to be alkaline forming. But forced stimulation of organs by drugs produces a lot of acid.

Drugs release hormones or adrenalin by stimulating

the adrenal glands. Cortical hormones and adrenalin increase glucose in the blood and one feels a high energy from the burning up of glucose. The result is a high production of acid. Therefore, taking drugs is like eating sugar. It requires a large amount of minerals to maintain the blood in an alkaline condition. Seaweeds are the best food for this.

The next common sickness among the drug takers is kidney weakness, which manifests in frequent urination, bladder troubles, rashes, skin troubles, tiredness in the back, mineral imbalance in the blood (which causes great sensitivity to excess salt intake), and autonomic nervous system imbalance. People with these problems must be careful of the amount of salt they take. Ginger fomentation on the back of the kidneys is often very good for the kidneys. Azuki beans and black beans are good to eat or drink their juice. Less drinking is recommended but too restricted drinking will cause weakness.

However, the best remedy for the kidneys is to work hard so that one will perspire at least once a day. Without physical activity, strengthening the kidneys takes a long time even if one eats macrobiotically. Of hard work, gardening with bare feet is best.

Lastly, the most difficult trouble among drug takers is one who has a damaged or weakened interbrain, which controls body homeostasis (body temperature, amount of oxygen, water, blood sugar, etc.). The interbrain is also the connecting junction between mental activity and physical activity; therefore, one who has damaged this area lacks coordination of these two activities. In other words, he may understand or speak very well about how to eat and what to do, but he can neither eat nor do as he says. I have met such young people so many times. They look healthy and sharp but they cannot practice what they preach. For them to stay on the diet is quite difficult. Therefore, they fool around with various diets. However, they can improve their condition if they wish to, although very slowly. In other words, without a clear and firm will to build health by oneself, no one can recover from the suffering caused by drug abuse. In order to acquire a firmer will to establish health, one needs to know how deep his sickness is. As long as he thinks he is healthy and good, he will not search out health, even though all his behavior indicates that he is searching. He is too ignorant, too arrogant, or has not suffered enough.

Macrobiotics is a useful and practical technique even for sickness resulting from drug abuse. However, without humility and great aspiration toward Real Self, it gives no help. Whoever wants to observe macrobiotics for their health must consider spiritual cultivation too.

5. Fatigue and Acidity

One of the main causes of fatigue is increased acidity in the blood. Overworking, overeating (especially overeating of acid forming foods such as meat and grains), constipation, diarrhea, kidney trouble, and liver trouble all lead to acidity of blood. This acid condition of the blood causes fatigue. Why?

Carbon dioxide is continually being formed in the body by the different intracellular metabolic processes. The carbon (C) contained in foods metabolizes to combine with oxygen to form carbon dioxide. This in turn diffuses into the intercellular fluids and blood, and is transported to the lungs where it diffuses into the alveoli and is transferred to the atmosphere by pulmonary ventilation. However, several minutes are required for this passage of carbon dioxide from the cells to the atmosphere. Since the carbon dioxide is not removed instantaneously, an average of 1.2 milliliters of dissolved carbon dioxide is normally in the extracellular fluids. This carbon dioxide combines with water and forms carbonic acid (H_2CO_3) which is yin. If carbon dioxide increases, carbonic acid (yin) increases. The hydrogen ion of the carbonic acid has a direct action on the respiratory center in the medulla oblongata, which controls breathing, causing increase in the rate of respiration (yin stimulates yang). However, this is only true when the blood is alkaline. If carbon dioxide in the blood increases too much as the result of overworking, overeating of meats, or bad circulation of blood, carbonic acid increases the level of blood acidity (yin). This blood acidity damages the respiratory center in the medulla oblongata and causes reduced breathing. The reduction in breathing causes less oxygen to be inhaled and results in less oxygen for cell metabolism. Fatigue is a result.

There are several ways of curing fatigue, depending on the cause of the fatigue:

1. Eating less and chewing well will be most important in the cure of all fatigue.

2. Improve blood circulation using:
   a. Hot foot bath or ginger compress on foot.
   b. Shower with alternately hot and cold water.
   c. Apply Dō-In massage.

3. Apply ginger compress over the kidney.

4. Drink shoyu-bancha (sho-ban), ume-sho bancha (salt plum, ginger, soy sauce, bancha tea). If this is too salty, drink plum concentrate tea (bainiku ekisu extract).

5. Eat plenty of salad, especially with green vegetables; eat pickles, etc.

6. Practice breathing exercises. In the Orient, breathing exercises developed as a means of curing fatigue and improving health.

 a. Yogic breathing exercise:
  Stand up and breathe deeply. Stop breathing and bend body down. Exhale and bring the upper body upright while holding the breath. Bend legs several times, then inhale. Repeat this exercise several times and fatigue will be relieved.

 b. Buddhist breathing exercise (Shin sect):
  Sit up and stretch out legs. Raise arms until they are horizontal. Inhale and hold breath. Bend upper body forward while stretching legs. Keep this posture as long as possible. Then bring the upper body back to starting position. Exhale. Repeat several times.

 Both breathing exercises are good for curing fatigue because they reduce carbon dioxide from the lungs and blood. The reduction of carbon dioxide makes the blood more alkaline and increases cell metabolism and stimulates the respiratory center to increase breathing.

7. Walking and any exercises are also good for fatigue when done in the proper amount. In modern society we tend to sit and not use the legs often enough. Walking or gardening in the early morning will be the best exercise and will result in a tireless body and a joyous and healthy life.

6. Acid and Alkaline and Mentality

An acidic condition inhibits nerve action and an alkaline condition stimulates nerve action. One who has an alkaline blood condition can think and act (decide) well. On the other hand, one who has an acidic blood condition cannot think well or act quickly, clearly, or decisively. Therefore, it is very important to maintain an alkaline blood condition all the time – not only for physical health, but also for mental awareness.

The diet is a great help in maintaining alkalinity of blood; however, it does not reveal results in a day or two. It takes a longer time to show the effect. For a long time I searched for a quick way to change an acidic to an alkaline condition. Finally, I found one through religious rituals. Japanese Shinto religion strongly recommends performing the misogi ritual, in which one takes a cold water bath or shower in a river, waterfall, or the ocean. One health advocate recommends taking an alternately hot and cold bath. A friend of mine did it, and I saw he was much better than before – physically and spiritually. Therefore, I started taking a cold shower every night after a hot bath. I realized the effect immediately. The cold shower made me very high spirited and gave better brain function. When I was craving some foods such as fish, the cold shower stopped it immediately. It creates tremendous will power and high judging ability. The reason for this lies in the fact that a cold shower makes the blood alkaline, while hot showers (baths) make the blood acid.

It is a good ritual. The Catholic and other Christian religions have the baptism ceremony and Shinto has the misogi ceremony. Making our blood alkaline, those ceremonies are excellent ways of improving our thinking ability and high spirit.

I recommend taking cold showers for anyone who has problems in his or her life or family; who has too much stress; or who wishes to improve his judgment – to attain a clearcut view on life and to know what to do.

The best time for this is at midnight or in the early morning. It is necessary to continue for about ten days in order to have some sign of improvement in thinking.

When taking a cold shower, don't take it from the head. Rather take it from the legs up – front, right shoulder, back, and left shoulder – turning clockwise – then, head last. One who has a weak heart should observe carefully and go easy.

7. Cancer and Acid and Alkaline

Alexis Carrel kept a chicken heart alive in an alkaline solution for twenty-eight years. He was able to do this by changing the solution every day; he maintained a certain proportion of elements so that the solution was always slightly alkaline. Also, acid byproducts of cell metabolism were eliminated by renewing the solution every day. The chicken heart died when Carrel stopped changing the solution.

According to modern physiology, this is true also for humans, as I mentioned previously. Our body cells are surrounded by fluids which should be slightly alkaline in order to sustain life. If you go jogging or do heavy exercise, you experience shortness of breath, tiredness, and muscle stiffness. This is the result of the production and accumulation of lactic acid, which is in turn the result of the incomplete combustion of glucose. In other words, under conditions of heavy exercise the body is not getting enough oxygen to metabolize glucose. At such times, the pH of the blood will be around 7.26 – 7.27 instead of the normal 7.3 - 7.4. This is an acidic condition of the blood. This kind of acidity is corrected by the body's buffering system, which changes strong acids to weak acids and elminates them as carbon dioxide (CO_2) which we exhale as part of our breath.

If the condition of our extracellular fluids, especially the blood, becomes acidic, our physical condition will first manifest tiredness, proneness to catching colds, etc. When these fluids become more acidic, our condition then manifests pains and suffering such as headache, chest pain, stomachache, etc. According to Keiichi Morishita in his *Hidden Truth of Cancer*, if the blood develops a more acidic condition, then our body inevitably deposits these excess acidic substances in some area of the body such so that the blood will be able to maintain an alkaline condition. As this tendency continues, such areas increase in acidity and some cells die; then these dead cells themselves turn into acids. However, some other cells may adapt in that environment. In other words, instead of dying - as normal cells do in an acid environment - some cells survive by becoming abnormal cells. These abnormal cells are called malignant cells. Malignant cells do not correspond with brain function nor with our own DNA memory code. Therefore, malignant cells grow indefinitely and without order. This is cancer.

One of the most common ways to cause an acidic condition of the body fluids is the over consumption of fat. Since fat does not dissolve in water, if one over consumes fatty foods all the time, chunks of undissolved fat float in the arteries to the capillaries. These chunks of fat clog the capillaries and stop the supply of nutrients and oxygen. Stopping the supply of nutrients and oxygen causes the death of the cells at the end of clogged capillaries. The dead cells turn to acid. The acidic condition of the body fluids causes normal cells to change to malignant cells as explained above. Cancer of the breast and of the colon are mostly caused by the consumption of too much fat.

Over consumption of protein causes an acidic condition because the excess protein breaks down and produces blood urea nitrogen. This urea causes the kidneys to excrete too much water, along with alkaline forming minerals. Thus, the over consumption of protein causes an acidic condition of the blood.

Other foods which cause an acidic condition of the body fluids are sugar, white rice, white flour, chemicals added to foods, medicinal drugs, and synthetic drugs. All those foods and drugs cause acidic conditions in two ways. On the one hand, they each contain acid forming elements, and on the other hand, not one of them contributes any balancing alkaline forming elements. So they not only produce acids; they also use up the body's alkaline forming elements to neutralize the acids which they produce.

Physiological conditions such as weak kidneys and constipation also cause an acidic condition of the body fluids. Body activities always produce acids such as sulphuric acid, acetic acid, and lactic acid. If the kidneys are weak, those acids cannot be eliminated and they cause acidic body fluid. In the case of constipation, the stool putrifies in the colon and increases acidic conditions in the body. In my opinion this is the beginning of colon cancer.

Why does an acidic condition in the body fluids cause cells to become malignant? Acidity in the extracellular fluids kills nerve cells which are connected with the brain, and acidity in the intracellular fluids damages cell nuclei, which control cellular growth. Therefore, cancer develops in the following stages:

1. Ingestion of many acid forming foods, fatty

foods, protein rich foods, refined foods, carcinogenic substances such as nitrites, and chemically treated foods in general. X-ray scans contribute even at this stage.

2. Increased constipation.
3. Increase of acidity in the blood. This causes an increase of white cells and a decrease of red cells, which is the beginning of leukemia.
4. Increase of acidity in the extracellular fluids.
5. Increase of acidity in the intracellular fluids.
6. Birth of malignant cells. This is the stage of cancer called initiation.
7. The further consumption of many yin foods. Receiving high levels of radiation, chemical, and drug treatment. This is the stage of cancer called promotion.

The above opinion on cancer development is my conclusion after studying the cancer research of several scientists. Dr. Yanagisawa observed the blood of two types of leukemia patients: 1. survivors of the atomic explosion on Hiroshima, and 2. a fisherman who suffered from atomic bomb radiation near the Bikini Island test site in the Pacific Ocean. He found that these patients had blood which was low in calcium and magnesium ions. Since both calcium and magnesium are alkaline forming elements, to be low in them is the same thing as having an acidic condition of the blood. In our body, red blood cells make up 10 mg. per 100 milliliters of serum. Normally, for every 100 mg. of calcium, 60 mg. are in crystal form and 40 mg. are calcium ions in solution. When the blood is healthy, the ratio of crystaline calcium to ionic calcium is 6 to 4. When one is sick or tired, the number of calcium ions decreases. In the case of the leukemia patients, when the number of calcium ions decreased to 15 mg. per 100 ml. of serum, the patients died. (From *Wheat Diet*, by Fumimasa Yanagisawa.)

According to *Cell Society*, by Dr. S. Okada, cancer cells grow well in a culture solution produced by the metabolic wastes of regular cells. Since the metabolic waste material of regular cells is acidic, cancer cells, then, like this acidic condition.

Therefore, to prevent the development of cancer or to stop cancer growth, the macrobiotic diet recommends not eating acid forming foods – especially sugar, animal foods (including fish and milk products), refined foods, or foods treated with chemical additives. Furthermore, macrobiotics recommends increasing blood circulation, kidney strength, and bowel movement.

Another macrobiotic recommendation comes from the yin and yang principle. Cancer cells grow quickly, indefinitely, and without order, and therefore are yin. Consequently, yin acid forming foods are the first things to eliminate from the diet. These foods are listed in Section II of Table 20 (p. 90); among these foods are sugar, drugs, and chemical additives, and they should be avoided above all else.

Although grains are also acid forming, they are yang and they neither cause nor promote cancer. Because grains are balanced in yin and yang and contain important vitamins, proteins, carbohydrates, fibers, and minerals, the macrobiotic diet recommends whole grains as the main foods for cancer patients, and with good results. Whole grains (acid forming) along with selected vegetables (alkaline forming), sea vegetables, and condiments – such as sea salt, miso, and authentic soy sauce (all alkaline forming) – make, to my knowledge, the best foods for both resisting and preventing cancer.

Cancer cells are very yin; even so-called yang cancer cells are very yin. Therefore, the macrobiotic diet prohibits fruits and some vegetables which are very yin, even if they are alkaline forming. However, for the prevention of cancer growth, not only yin but also yang foods (all animal foods, fish and dairy foods) are prohibited. Why? First of all, these are acid forming; secondly, they are rich in protein and fat. Both protein and fat are acid forming; in addition, protein helps cancer cells grow because cells are made of protein.

Generally speaking, cancer grows when sugar and animal foods are consumed together, the latter supplying both protein to form cancer cells and fat to cause constipation and bad circulation. The sugar supplies energy to grow. Taken separately, protein and sugar are not so harmful. For instance, Eskimos consume a lot of animal foods but not much sugar, and they do not have many cancer cases. In India, on the other hand, people consume much sugar but not much meat, and there are not many cancer cases there either.

Cancer causing foods are a combination of the following:

Very yin, acid forming foods such as:

Sugar, saccharin, or vinegar.
Chemical additives, colorings, and
    preservatives.
Canned foods.
Highly processed or refined foods.

Yang, acid forming foods such as:

All meats—chicken, beef, pork, and fish.
Dairy products.

Very yin, alkaline forming foods such as:

> All fruits and fruit juices.
> Potato, tomato, eggplant, asparagus,
>   avocado, spinach, and beets. (See Section I
>   of Table 20, p. 91).

In conclusion, in order to either stop or prevent cancer growth, my advice is as follows:

1. Stop the consumption of sugar and animal food, fruits, milk and dairy products.
2. Avoid beans except two to three times per month, and then eat only azuki beans.
3. Completely avoid chemical and refined foods.
4. Eat meals which are comprised of 50-60% whole grains and 25-35% vegetables and sea vegetables.
5. Eat one or two cups of macrobiotic miso soup every day.
6. Drink yang, alkaline forming beverages – mu tea, yannoh, ohsawa coffee, and bancha tea.
7. Use only natural, authentic condiments such as miso, soy sauce, gomashio, tekka, umeboshi, etc.
8. Cook according to the season, weather, and the individual constitution.
9. Practice deep breathing, singing, or chanting, but not heavy exercise such as jogging.
10. If a person is heavy and/or fat, take a sauna every day. If skinny, take one every other day. A dry sauna is better than a wet sauna.
11. A cold shower is recommended to alkalize the blood and other body fluids.
12. Cook with gas instead of electricity.

8. Conclusion

Nature manifests the two antagonistic yet complementary powers in plants, animals, and things everywhere. The ancient Chinese wise men called these manifestations yin and yang. Modern science calls them positive and negative, plus and minus, electron and proton, expansion and contraction, induction and deduction, man and woman, male and female, and acid and alkaline.

Where do acid and alkaline come from? What is their origin? If you understand this, you can see an entirely different view of this world.

There is a Zen koan: "What is the sound of one hand?" Two hands create sound. Clapping cannot be created by only one hand. Zen students must answer this. In the same way, you cannot see the origin of acid and alkaline. What you see or taste is everything manifesting either as acid or alkaline. The origin of acid and alkaline is where there is no acid and alkaline – that is to say, where there is no sound, no light, no movement, no color, no hot, no cold, no acid, no alkaline, no left, no right, no old, no young, no pain, no joy. . . . Buddhists call it *ku*, Taoists call it *mu*, Shintoists call it *kami*. This is the origin of acid and alkaline. Foods are carriers of these two forces, and eating food we produce antagonistic and complementary cells, muscles, nerves, hormones, enzymes, genes, organs, and thoughts.

Since our life is the manifestation of two forces, our actions, living, and thoughts always have antagonism and contradiction. However, if there is antagonism, there should exist complementarity. Therefore, the most important lesson to learn from acid and alkaline is to accept an antagonism whenever you come across it, and turn it to complementarity in your life.

This is the real balancing of acid and alkaline.

Bibliography

Aihara, Cornellia – *The Calendar Cookbook*, GOMF, Oroville, 1979.

Aihara, Cornellia and Herman – *The Dō of Cooking*, GOMF, Oroville, 1982.

Bowes and Church – *Food Values of Portions Commonly Used*, J. B. Lippincott Co., Philadelphia, 1970.

Cannon, Dr. Walter – *The Wisdom of the Body*, W. W. Norton & Co., New York, rev. ed., 1939.

Carque, Otto – *Vital Facts About Foods*, Natural Brands, Los Angeles, 1933.

Carrel, Alexis – *Man, The Unknown, Harper, New York, 1935*.

Chishima, Kikuo – Revolution of Biology and Medicine, Vol. 9, Neo-Haematological Society Press, Gifu, Japan, 1972.

Collier's Encyclopedia – Macmillan Educational Corporation, New York, 1979.

Encyclopedia Britannica – Chicago, 1974.

Engels, Frederick – *Dialectics of Nature*, International Publishers, New York, 1940.

Goth, Andres, M. D. – *Medical Pharmacology*, C. V. Mosby Co., 1976.

Guyton, Arthur, M. D. – *Function of the Human Body*, W. B. Saunders Co., Philadelphia, 1959. Reprint 1969.

Guyton, Arthur, M. D. – *Textbook of Medical Physiology*, W. B. Saunders Co., Philadelphia, 1956.

Ions, Veronica – *Indian Mythology*, Hamlyn Publishing Group LTD, London, 1967.

Ishizuka, Sagen – *Foods for Longevity* (1898), Nippon Centre Ignoramus, Tokyo.

Ishizuka, Sagen – *Scientific Diet for Longevity,* Haku Bunkan, Tokyo, (1896 o/p).

Jackson, Robert G., M. D. – *How to be Always Well,* Printcraft Limited, Toronto, 1932.

Katase, Dr. Tan – *Calcium Medicine,* Ningen No Igaku Co., Osaka, 1948.

Moon, J. Y. – *Macrobiotic Explanation of Pathological Calcification,* GOMF, Oroville, 1974.

Morishita, Keiichi, *The Hidden Truth of Cancer,* GOMF, Oroville, 1976.

Morse, J., ed., *Funk & Wagnalls Encyclopedia, Vol. I,* Reader's Digest Books, Inc., New York, 1969.

Ohsawa, George – *Practical Guide to Far Eastern Macrobiotic Medicine,* GOMF, San Francisco, 1973.

Ohsawa, George – *The Book of Judgment,* GOMF, Oroville, 1980.

Ohsawa, George – *The Unique Principle,* GOMF, Oroville, 1976.

Ohsawa, George – *Zen Macrobiotics,* Ohsawa Foundation, Los Angeles, 1965.

Okada, Tokindo – *Saiko No Shakai (Cell Society),* Kodansha, Tokyo, 1972.

Pinsent, John – *Greek Mythology,* Hamlyn Publishing Group LTD, London, 1969.

Quarton, Melnichuck and Schmidt, eds. – *Neurosciences: A Study Program,* Rockefeller University Press, New York, 1967.

U. S. Department of Agriculture – *Composition of Foods*, Washington, D. C., 1963.

U. S. Government Printing Office, Washington D. C. – *The Yearbook of Agriculture, 1959*.

Williams and Lansford, eds. – *The Encyclopedia of Biochemistry*, Reinhold Publishing Corp., New York, 1967.

Yanagisawa, Dr. Fumimasa – *Wheat for Health*, Yomiuri Press, Tokyo, 1975.

Acknowledgment is given for the kind permission granted by the publishers from whose works selections have been used or reprinted in this book. The following credit lines are included as requested:

Selection is reprinted from THE WISDOM OF THE BODY by Walter B. Cannon, M.D. by permission of W. W. Norton & Company, Inc. Copyright 1932 by Walter B. Cannon. Copyright renewed 1960 by Cornelia J. Cannon. Revised Edition copyright 1939 by Walter B. Cannon. Renewed 1968 1967 by Cornelia J. Cannon.

From THE ENCYCLOPEDIA OF BIOCHEMISTRY, edited by Roger J. Williams and Edwin M. Lansford, Jr. © 1967 by Litton Educational Publishing, Inc. Reprinted by permission of Van Nostrand Reinhold Co.

Reprinted with permission from *Collier's Encyclopedia*. © 1979 Macmillan Educational Corporation.

From "Alkaloids" in *Encyclopaedia Britannica*, 15th edition (1974).

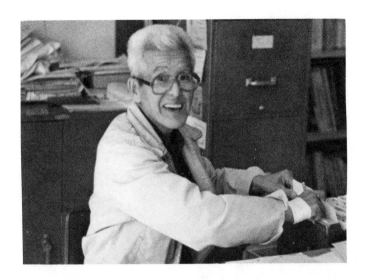

Herman Aihara was born in Arita (Saga Prefecture), a small town in southern Japan, in September of 1920. He was adopted into an uncle's home due to the poverty conditions of his large family.

He was accepted into the School of Engineering at the reputable Waseda University, and in 1942 he graduated from the University with a bachelor's degree in Metallurgical Engineering.

Before entering the University he had heard George Ohsawa at a lecture and became very interested in the study of yin and yang. After the War, he attended Ohsawa's classes and eventually decided to emigrate to the United States to teach macrobiotics.

He worked with Michio Kushi to establish macrobiotics in New York from 1952 to 1961 and was elected the first president of the Ohsawa Foundation in New York. After moving to California, he was elected president of the Ohsawa Foundation in Los Angeles in 1969. He founded and became president of the George Ohsawa Macrobiotic Foundation in San Francisco in 1970, and moved GOMF to Oroville, California in 1974.

Mr. Aihara is continuously active in research and study along with writing, translating, lecturing, and giving personal consultations in the United States and abroad.

121